Advanced Vaginal Surgery

Advanced Vaginal Surgery

Shirish S Sheth MD FRCOG (Ad Eundem) FACOG (Hon)
FACS FICS FCPS FICOG FAMS FSOGC (Hon)

Hon. Professor, Obstetrician and Gynecologist
King Edward Memorial Hospital and Seth GS Medical College, Mumbai, Maharashtra, India (1964–1994)
President, International Federation of Gynecology and Obstetrics (FIGO) from 2000–2003
Consultant Gynecologist: Breach Candy and Saifee Hospitals, Mumbai, Maharashtra, India

Carl W Zimmerman MD

Division Director
Female Pelvic Medicine and Reconstructive Surgery
Frances and John C. Burch Chair in Obstetrics and Gynecology
Vanderbilt University School of Medicine
Nashville, Tennessee, USA

Seth Finkelstein MD FACOG FPMRS

Lenox Hill Hospital, Manhattan
Kingsbrook Jewish Medical Center, Brooklyn
New York, USA

Foreword

Prof Alan D Hewson

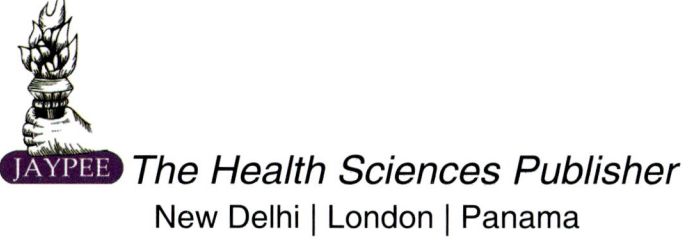

JAYPEE *The Health Sciences Publisher*
New Delhi | London | Panama

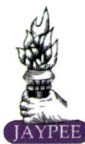

Jaypee Brothers Medical Publishers (P) Ltd

Headquarters

Jaypee Brothers Medical Publishers (P) Ltd.
4838/24, Ansari Road, Daryaganj
New Delhi 110 002, India
Phone: +91-11-43574357
Fax: +91-11-43574314
E-mail: jaypee@jaypeebrothers.com

Overseas Offices

J.P. Medical Ltd.
83, Victoria Street, London
SW1H 0HW (UK)
Phone: +44-20 3170 8910
Fax: +44(0)20 3008 6180
E-mail: info@jpmedpub.com

Jaypee-Highlights Medical Publishers Inc.
City of Knowledge, Bld. 235, 2nd Floor, Clayton
Panama City, Panama
Phone: +1 507-301-0496
Fax: +1 507-301-0499
E-mail: cservice@jphmedical.com

Jaypee Brothers Medical Publishers (P) Ltd.
17/1-B, Babar Road, Block-B, Shaymali
Mohammadpur, Dhaka-1207
Bangladesh
Mobile: +08801912003485
E-mail: jaypeedhaka@gmail.com

Jaypee Brothers Medical Publishers (P) Ltd.
Bhotahity, Kathmandu, Nepal
Phone: +977-9741283608
E-mail: kathmandu@jaypeebrothers.com

Website: www.jaypeebrothers.com
Website: www.jaypeedigital.com

© 2017, Jaypee Brothers Medical Publishers

The views and opinions expressed in this book are solely those of the original contributor(s)/author(s) and do not necessarily represent those of editor(s) of the book.

All rights reserved. No part of this publication may be reproduced, stored or transmitted in any form or by any means, electronic, mechanical, photocopying, recording or otherwise, without the prior permission in writing of the publishers.

All brand names and product names used in this book are trade names, service marks, trademarks or registered trademarks of their respective owners. The publisher is not associated with any product or vendor mentioned in this book.

Medical knowledge and practice change constantly. This book is designed to provide accurate, authoritative information about the subject matter in question. However, readers are advised to check the most current information available on procedures included and check information from the manufacturer of each product to be administered, to verify the recommended dose, formula, method and duration of administration, adverse effects and contraindications. It is the responsibility of the practitioner to take all appropriate safety precautions. Neither the publisher nor the author(s)/editor(s) assume any liability for any injury and/or damage to persons or property arising from or related to use of material in this book.

This book is sold on the understanding that the publisher is not engaged in providing professional medical services. If such advice or services are required, the services of a competent medical professional should be sought.

Every effort has been made where necessary to contact holders of copyright to obtain permission to reproduce copyright material. If any have been inadvertently overlooked, the publisher will be pleased to make the necessary arrangements at the first opportunity.

Inquiries for bulk sales may be solicited at: jaypee@jaypeebrothers.com

Advanced Vaginal Surgery

First Edition: **2017**
ISBN: 978-93-5270-017-2
Printed at Sanat Printers.

Dedicated to

All those who have contraindication, reluctance and tension
All those who have made mistakes as I have,
All those who are enthusiastic, desirous and ambitious to learn,
promote the least and invasive Vaginal Hysterectomy,
All those who will increase their grace and share the exciting surgery
through lacunae-n-skill, loopholes-n-complications to coming generations in the best interests of women.

Foreword

It is a privilege to introduce this latest addition to the gynecological literature by that master vaginal surgeon, Professor Shirish S Sheth and his two collaborators. My own love affair with vaginal hysterectomy began in 1956 working as a registrar to an Oxford trained gynecologist in Hobart in Tasmania, so I have had the opportunity to see a dramatic change in attitude over the last 60 years. At that time, the vast majority of hysterectomies world-wide were done abdominally through a midline incision, and the change in approach was extremely slow. Working in Oxford in 1957-58, I was part of the trailblazing "Oxford 1000" vaginal hysterectomy series reported by Hawksworth and Roux, who building on the Bonney/Stallworthy heritage documented outstanding results, and altered forever the resistance to change in the United Kingdom. The campaign was continued later by Mohammed Hefni, Adam Magos and Ray Garry with major contributions to the literature. Across the Atlantic, Heaney in Chicago from the 1940s and many other innovators were spreading the same message, and Joel Cohen from South Africa, later at Beilinson in Tel Aviv, stood out as another prophet proclaiming the vaginal hysterectomy message. Australian gynecologists at that time virtually all trained in the UK, and made pilgrimages to centers like Oxford where vaginal hysterectomy was becoming an art form and brought the techniques back to this country, presumably the reason why vaginal hysterectomy rates here are the highest in the developed world. Another innovator in the USA was James Ingram in Tampa, whose associates Hoffman and Spellacy's book on the Difficult Vaginal Hysterectomy in 1995 became a classic, and proponents of day stay vaginal hysterectomy like Summitt in 1993 gave another new message. The brilliant contributions of Professor David Nichols from Providence Rhode Island with his Thanksgiving weekend workshops will also never be forgotten. Of course there were others of prominence, but the emerging contributions of Professor Sheth from the early 1990s with his demonstration that adnexal surgery at vaginal hysterectomy could be both feasible and safe, greatly expanding its role, was a revelation to most gynecologists. His unique gifts as a superb technical operator, gifted teacher, and one with the courage to go where none had gone before has ensured his place at the pinnacle of our profession. Astonishingly he has been able to combine a massive operative workload, and charitable work with onerous responsibilities in the highest echelons of our discipline internationally. As hysterectomy rates worldwide are steadily falling associated with newer modalities of nonsurgical treatment, it is highly likely that his enormous experience in this field will never be matched, so this new book is even more important for posterity. I see this volume as the culmination of his life's work emphasizing yet again the enormous potential scope and utility of the vaginal approach to pelvic disease, complemented by contributions from two other experienced vaginal surgeons. It is aimed at experienced operators, but should be on the shelf of any gynecologist who genuinely wishes to know the potential of our discipline in the 21st century and who wishes be part of informed debate on the challenges of advanced vaginal surgery.

Prof Alan D Hewson AM PhD MD FRANZCOG FRACS FRCOG FRCSEd
Conjoint Professor, Faculty of Health,
University of Newcastle, NSW, Australia

Preface

When evidence-based studies show that vaginal is the choicest route for hysterectomy keeping abdomen intact, one wonders that why cannot same be utilized for much more than hysterectomy. The major focus is on the best surgical practices, keeping away greater invasion, have minimum hospital stay, complications, and cost, etc.

As experience of vaginal surgery increases, indications for it can also increase by a corresponding decrease in the related contraindications. This can make one to advance in selectively performed vaginal hysterectomy with or without salpingo-oophorectomy to greater heights. Authors have tried to bring to surface the strategies and techniques to conquer and achieve what is usually considered as impossible or taken for granted as a contraindication. We present our favorable experience for the colleagues to get familiar and consider the possibility of going beyond routine and give several advantages to the suffering patients. The contents of the book include vast majority of clinical conditions met commonly in practice but willingness to utilize such opportunities to promote professional judgment and implement beyond routine is uncommon to rare.

Safety and success in the operating room depend on: (a) comfort with surgical anatomy, (b) setting a strategy preoperatively, (c) the willingness to re-evaluate the same intraoperatively and exercise good clinical judgment—readers will repeatedly find these concepts discussed in this text within the presented cases.

Gynecologists, particularly vaginal hysterectomists, need to look beyond by gradually marching and mastering the art of vaginal surgery without laparoscopic assistance. No doubt, laparoscopic surgery has opened the door for competitive aspects and attempt to perform what is in the best interests for the patient.

Some of the contraindications are related to lackings in the past and are well suited to the surgeon's convenience and/or weakness. In the past, there were no ultrasonography, MRI or CT scans, tumor markers, laparoscope and strong antibiotics. In fact, contraindications like uterine size greater than 12–14 weeks or the presence of mobile benign ovarian cyst were in the best interests of all the learners to prevent complications but as we indulge in practice, we gather experience to override the situation and realize that some of these contraindications can be reduced or omitted. Conditions like nulliparity, uterine fibroid(s), and previous abdominopelvic surgery, particularly caesarean delivery, are iatrogenic and not genuine contraindications, but easy excuses to open the abdomen and perform easy hysterectomy or unscientifically promote laparoscopic hysterectomy and take away the focus on the vaginal route and its advantages.

Despite intra-abdominal mess or grossly pathological situation with disturbing findings, does one not approach abdomen for the abdominal surgery and override the situation or does one rule out abdominal route for hysterectomy? Similarly, we should heavily respect the God-given vaginal route.

Examination under anesthesia should become the gold standard to confirm the route and technique because it confirms, convinces and guides. Laparoscopic surgery is a boon and a great addition to our armamentarium as it has demonstrated the superiority of the vaginal over the abdominal route beyond an iota of doubt. The biggest advantage of laparoscopic hysterectomy is that it prevents opening of the abdomen. However, it cannot replace or compete with vaginal hysterectomy when both are possible. In actuality, vaginal hysterectomy is the least invasive, less invasive than the so-called minimally invasive laparoscopic hysterectomy and the God-given natural orifice leading to natural route. However, uncommonly, a look inside the peritoneal cavity can change the picture and this can be achieved by a single puncture of 5 mm diagnostic laparoscopy. One must also note that 80% of the world is without laparoscope and/or laparoscopists. Therefore, if one does not advance in vaginal hysterectomy and beyond, innumerable abdomens will be opened.

If vaginal surgery was marketed with the advantage of abdomen remaining virgin or scarless, certainly in a consumer-driven society, goods, i.e. vaginal, would have been more in demand.

Surgical practice will get added attraction and affinity if vaginal hysterectomy is promoted for women with endometrial cancer, who do not require lymphadenectomy. Schauta's radical vaginal hysterectomy with laparoscopic lymphadenectomy in cases of invasive cancer of the cervix can really spare the opening of the abdomen. However, we need gynecologists performing Schauta's radical hysterectomy to invite laparoscopic lymphadenectomy, spare the abdomen and promote laparoscopic surgery.

Shirish S Sheth
Carl W Zimmerman
Seth Finkelstein

Acknowledgments

For undertaking difficult or contraindicated cases, one may need high cader anesthesiologists and for which we are thankful to par excellence display by Anesthesiologists Dr Shilpa Bhojraj, Dr D Dasgupta, Dr Daizy Jokhi, Dr Hemant Mehta, Dr Amla Rege, Dr Shaila Telang and others. Similarly to colleague physicians Dr M Jain, Dr S Golwala, Dr Bharat Shah and others. We are equally thankful to assistance received from Dr Sudeshna Ray and expert nurses Mrs EP Lobo and Mrs Aleyamma Jose. Many thanks to reassuring Dr Kurush Paghdiwalla for his availability/standby, if laparoscopic surgery or complicated surgery was required.

We wish to sincerely thank all the contributors and gratefully acknowledge the assistance and given credit to Ms Kavita Dama and Mrs Rita Chettiar for the laborious work on computer.

Lastly, we also thank Shri Jitendar P Vij (Group Chairman), Mr Ankit Vij (Group President), Ms Chetna Malhotra Vohra (Associate Director–Content Strategy), and Ms Nedup Denka Bhutia (Development Editor) of Jaypee Brothers Medical Publishers, New Delhi, India, for giving us a go-ahead at the very beginning and helping us in every way possible to bring out this book. As always, we are deeply indebted to those authors and editors who have labored to write this book without much effort.

Contents

Section 1: Vaginal Hysterectomy with Uterine Debulking

Introduction   3
- CASE 1: Vaginal Hysterectomy (VH) with Uterine Debulking   8
- CASE 2: Vaginal Hysterectomy (VH) with Uterine Debulking Plus Bilateral Salpingo-oophorectomy (BSO) (CA125: 516)   9
- CASE 3: Vaginal Hysterectomy with Uterine Debulking Plus Ovarian Cystectomy   10
- CASE 4: Vaginal Hysterectomy with Massive Uterine Debulking Plus Bilateral Salpingo-oophorectomy (Right Hydrosalpinx)   11
- CASE 5: Vaginal Hysterectomy with Debulking Plus Bilateral Salpingo-oophorectomy with H/O Two Caesarean Sections   13
- CASE 6: Vaginal Hysterectomy with Uterine Debulking Plus Bilateral Salpingo-oophorectomy and Laparoscopic Cholecystectomy   14
- CASE 7: Nullipara: Large Debulking and Adnexectomy   17
- CASE 8: Nullipara and Obese: Debulking with Bilateral Salpingectomy   19
- CASE 9: Massive Debulking of Kilogram Uterus with Bilateral Salpingectomy-1   20
- CASE 10: Massive Debulking of Kilogram Uterus with Bilateral Salpingectomy-2   21
- CASE 11: Debulking of Large Adenomyoma, Bilateral Salpingectomy-1   22
- CASE 12: Debulking of Large Adenomyoma, Bilateral Salpingectomy-2   23
- CASE 13: Large Debulking with Bilateral Salpingectomy for Recurrent Postmenopause Bleeding   24
- CASE 14: Early Debulking with the Aid of Vasopressin   25

Section 2A: Vaginal Hysterectomy with History of Caesarean Section(s)

Introduction   29
- CASE 15: VH with Left Ovarian Cystectomy   30
- CASE 16: VH Plus Stress Urinary Incontinence (SUI) Repair   32
- CASE 17: VH with Uterine Debulking   33
- CASE 18: VH with Right Ovarian Cystectomy Plus ?Endometrial Hyperplasia   34
- CASE 19: VH with Left Salpingo-oophorectomy for Ovarian Endometrial Cyst in a Morbidly Obese Patient   35
- CASE 20: VH with BSO for Right Ovarian Endometriotic Cyst   37
- CASE 21: VH with BSO for Abnormal Uterine Bleeding (AUB) with History of Caesarean Sections and Rupture Uterus   39
- CASE 22: VH Plus Vaginal Cuff with BSO for Postmenopausal Bleeder in a Morbidly Obese and Diabetic Patient   41
- CASE 23: VH with Altered Approach to Vesicouterine Peritoneum (VUP)   42
- CASE 24: VH in Heavy Cigarette Smoker with H/O Two Classical Caesarean Sections via Midline Vertical Laparotomy   46
- CASE 25: VH with Uterine Debulking Plus Bilateral Salpingectomy of Tubal Remnants after Four Caesarean Sections and No Vaginal Births   47
- CASE 26: VH Plus Bilateral Salpingectomy after One Caesarean and No Vaginal Births   48
- CASE 27: VH with Uterine Debulking after Six Midline Vertical Laparotomies (Five Caesarean Sections and One Ectopic Pregnancy) in a Morbidly Obese Cigarette Smoker   49

Section 2B: Vaginal Hysterectomy with History of Uterine Surgery in Past

- CASE 28: VH in Nullipara with H/O Abdominal Myomectomy   53
- CASE 29: VH Plus Salpingectomy in Primipara with H/O Abdominal Myomectomy and Recurrent Large Fibroids   54

Section 3: Vaginal Hysterectomy with Adnexal Pathology

Introduction	57
CASE 30: VH with BSO for Large Bilateral Hydrosalpinx	60
CASE 31: VH with Left Salpingo-oophorectomy for Ovarian Endometrial Cyst in Morbidly Obese with Past History of Two Caesarean Sections	62
CASE 32: VH with BSO for Left Ovarian Endometrial Cyst and Right Ovarian Teratoma with H/O Two Caesarean Sections	64
CASE 33: VH with BSO for Bilateral Ovarian Endometrial Cysts with Positive "Dimple Sign"	66
CASE 34: VH with BSO for a Solid Ovarian Tumor	68
CASE 35: VH with BSO for ?Endometrial Polyp with an Ovarian Solid Tumor	69
CASE 36: VH with BSO followed by Laparotomy for Ovarian Cyst (Failed "Trial Vaginal Route" because of Ovarian "CA")	70
CASE 37: VH with BSO and Right Broad Ligament Myomectomy for Right Broad Ligament Fibroid (BLF)	71
CASE 38: VH with BSO for Twisted Left Ovarian Cyst	73

Section 4: Nullipara and Vaginal Hysterectomy

CASE 39: VH in Nullipara with Intact Hymen	77
CASE 40: VH with Uterine Debulking	79
CASE 41: VH with Uterine Debulking Plus Right Ovarian Endometrial Cystectomy (H/O Myomectomy)	80
CASE 42: VH with BSO for Bilateral Large Hydrosalpinx	81
CASE 43: VH Plus Vaginal Cuff with BSO in Obese, Diabetic with Endometrial Cancer	82
CASE 44: VH with BSO for Twisted Left Ovarian Cyst	83

Section 5: Vaginal Hysterectomy for Endometrial Cancer

Introduction	87
CASE 45: VH Plus Vaginal Cuff with BSO: Postmenopausal Bleeder with Endometrial Complex Hyperplasia with Atypia	91
CASE 46: VH Plus Vaginal Cuff with BSO: Postmenopausal Bleeder with Corpus Cancer Syndrome for Endometrial Cancer (CA)	93
CASE 47: VH Plus Vaginal Cuff with BSO for Endometrial CA	95
CASE 48: VH Plus Vaginal Cuff with BSO: Postmenopausal Bleeder with Corpus Cancer Syndrome. Failed "Trial Vaginal Route". Abdominal Surgery for LNR for Endometrial CA	96
CASE 49: VH Plus Vaginal Cuff with BSO for Endometrial Complex Hyperplasia with Atypia. Corpus CA Syndrome Plus a History of Cardiac Bypass	98
CASE 50: VH Plus Vaginal Cuff with BSO for Well-differentiated Endometrial Adenocarcinoma	99
CASE 51: VH Plus Vaginal Cuff with BSO: Postmenopausal Bleeder with Endometrial CA with History of Two Caesarean Sections Followed by Incisional Hernia Repair	100
CASE 52: VH Plus Vaginal Cuff with BSO Plus Laparoscopic Cholecystectomy for Postmenopausal Bleeder with Multiple Gallstones	101
CASE 53: Laparoscopic Cholecystectomy and VH Plus Vaginal Cuff with BSO: "Failed Trial Vaginal Route Case" Abdominal LNR for Endometrial CA	102

Section 6: Failed Trial Vaginal Hysterectomy/Trial Vaginal Route

CASE 54: Undiagnosed Uteroabdominal Band	107
CASE 55: Uterocervical Adhesions with Abdominal Wall	108
CASE 56: Diminished "Uterus-free" Space (Altered Uterocervical Angle)	110
CASE 57: Ovarian Endometriosis with Positive "Dimple Sign"	111
CASE 58: Large-sized Uterus	112
CASE 59: Ovarian Malignancy	113

CASE 60: Uterine Bulk Impedes Descent — 115
CASE 61: Extensive Adhesions from PID (Pelvic Inflammatory Disease) Limits Descent for VH — 116
CASE 62: Unanticipated Uterine Adhesions to Abdominal Wall-1 — 117
CASE 63: Unanticipated Uterine Adhesions to Abdominal Wall-2 — 118
CASE 64: Unanticipated Uterine Adhesions to Abdominal Wall-3 — 119
CASE 65: Parasitic Myoma and Inaccessible Adnexa Leads to Laparoscopic Completion of VH — 120

Section 7: Special Cases: Vaginal Hysterectomy

CASE 66: VH Plus H/O Rupture Uterus and Two Caesarean Sections — 123
CASE 67: VH Plus Broad Ligament Myomectomy without Laparoscopy Plus Contralateral Endometriotic Cyst — 125
CASE 68: VH for CIN III — 126
CASE 69: VH for Metastatic Breast Cancer Plus Uterine Adenomyosis — 127
CASE 70: VH: Prophylactic for Hydatidiform Mole — 128
CASE 71: VH with BSO for Twisted Ovarian Cyst — 129
CASE 72: VH for Uterine Fibroids with H/O Failed Abdominal Hysterectomy — 130
CASE 73: VH under Local Anesthesia for Pulmonary Fibrosis — 132
CASE 74: VH with Altered Approach to VUP (VH with BSO) — 134
CASE 75: VH with Bicornuate Uterus — 135
CASE 76: Bladder Stone Removal at VH Plus Anterior and Posterior Repair — 136
CASE 77: Vaginal Hysterectomy as Emergency Procedure for Cornual Ectopic Pregnancy — 138
CASE 78: Vaginal Supracervical Hysterectomy 10 Years after Mesh Hysteropexy — 139
CASE 79: Vaginal Hysterectomy (VH): Incarcerated Prolapse due to Cervical Leiomyoma and an Intramural Myoma — 140
CASE 80: VH in Nullipara with Ongoing Chemotherapy for Non-gynecologic Malignancies — 141
CASE 81: VH for Endometrial Carcinoma in Morbidly Obese with History of Caesarean Section — 142

Index — *143*

Introduction

All the cases given in Book are from the private or hospital practices of the authors. Each case is not 'a case report' but one out of such several that they have operated vaginally. Exceptions are five rare cases (1) History of rupture uterus and two Caesarean sections in past, (2) Nullipara with twisted ovarian cyst, (3) Removal of bladder stones, (4) Cornual pregnancy and (5) Large cervical fibroid. They all were operated vaginally for hysterectomy without use of laparoscope. Rest of all the cases are easily encountered in day-to-day practice and it is up to our experience, zeal and enthusiasm to attempt vaginally or otherwise. Minor variations in pelvic findings and operative steps will occur. Normal systemic findings are not mentioned and any abnormal are not omitted.

Indeed, for authors it is so satisfying to be together with same objectives despite vast geographical distance. We three respect, admire and stretch ourselves to utilize vaginal route as and when we can. We learn from perseverance and even failure to give benefits to our patients. Style of presentation will vary from Indian which hails from Britisher's era to American.

Book classically proves that where there is will there is way. 'Will' was to give the least invasion and big advantage to suffering women and 'way' was gynecological, i.e. vaginal route.

It is operator's keenness that accentuated to advance heavily in the field and to deal with contraindicated cases, overcome those contraindications and even convert some of them as indications to help suffering women.

We hope that readers get inspired and implement it someday, after acquiring back-up experience.

GENERAL INVASION

Vaginal hysterectomy (VH) is less invasive when compared with abdominal access either by opening the abdomen or by laparoscopic surgery. As far as just hysterectomy is concerned, abdominal or laparoscopic, the amount of cutting/severance is the same as for hysterectomy performed vaginally but there is additional surgery for opening of the abdomen or 4 to 5 through and through cuts from the skin to the peritoneal cavity respectively. It is common sense that abdominal cuts, large or small ones, are additional surgery and therefore makes laparoscopic hysterectomy (LH) or laparoscopically assisted vaginal hysterectomy (LAVH) more *invasive* than vaginal hysterectomy though labeled as minimally invasive. It is important to note that VH is the *'least'* invasive and laparoscopic hysterectomy is less invasive than abdominal hysterectomy (AH).

Unlike laparoscopic hysterectomy, instruments used for VH are almost permanent. Commercially, most of the instruments are used again and again for generations and do not require to be replaced after countless usage.

An intact abdomen permits rapid recovery, a shorter hospital stay with mental peace and is most economical. (Rest is our creation for gossip and/or commercial purpose). Thus with vaginal hysterectomy, woman will have the least invasive surgery and an intact abdomen. For the place of vaginal hysterectomy, answer will come from cochrane database and evidence-base conclusions as follows:

COCHRANE DATABASE REVIEW OF EVIDENCE-BASED HYSTERECTOMY STUDIES

- When VH is not feasible, LH may avoid the need for AH.
- No advantages of LH over VH could be found.
- VH with better outcomes and fewer complications than laparoscopic/TAH.
- Robotic H (RH) should either be abandoned or further evaluated.

In 2009, the American College of Obstetricians and Gynaecologists Committee concluded that the vaginal route is associated with better outcomes and fewer complications than the laparoscopic or abdominal hysterectomy.

Dr Harry Reich who pioneered or gave the first laparoscopic hysterectomy in 1989 recommended vaginal hysterectomy when it can be safely carried out in preference to laparoscopic hysterectomy.

There is no iota of doubt, that vaginal hysterectomy is the choicest in the best interests of suffering women. When indicated, not performing or offering it, only exposes the operator's weakness. Laparoscopic hysterectomy should be considered as an alternative to abdominal hysterectomy.

FOR GOING BEYOND ROUTINE VAGINAL HYSTERECTOMY: ATTEND TO FOLLOWING WITH CARE AND CONCERN

1. Detailed history.
2. Careful clinical examination.
3. At consultation, if indecisive findings for the vaginal route, examine her in super flexion position.
4. Clinically uterine size and sonographic uterine volume.
5. Reliable sonologist and sonography.
6. Examination under anesthesia (EUA).
7. Experienced anesthesiologist to maintain BP around 100–110/70–80 unless patient's system demands higher.
8. Experienced assistants.
9. Back up experience.
10. Consider trial VH and/or trial vaginal route. Confirm availability of laparoscopic assistance and/or laparotomy.
11. Self-confidence and perseverance, but within safety and one's own limit.

TO KEEP IN MIND

- Vascularity.
- Debulking.
- To sever available higher lateral connections.
- If not contraindicated by bleeding or risk of trauma, etc. persevere.
- To clamp popping out tube and ovary. It indicates that side's cornu is nearer to access.
- With history of Caesarean section, uncommon possibility of existence of an abdominal band from abdominal wall to anterior uterine surface, different from the dense adhesions between lower abdominal wall and uterocervical surface which gives the positive 'cervico-fundal sign'.
- Fundus held by or adherent to intestines/colon.
- To empty overful bladder intraoperatively particularly for adnexectomy (if surgery is prolonged).
- Better to stop and reevaluate, when required.
- Safer to abandon '*trial*' rather than have a complication, i.e. failed trial VH/vaginal route.
- Litigation.

ROLE OF PREOPERATIVE WORK UP

1. Investigations for operative fitness
2. Reliable sonography report
3. Hospital as per the patient's need
4. Select anesthesiologist(s), as required
5. Assisting surgeons (Residents/Nurses)
6. Frozen HP facility
7. Trial VH/Trial vaginal route
8. Standby laparoscopic surgeon's availability.

TRIAL VAGINAL HYSTERECTOMY: WHEREIN 'TRIAL' IS FOR THE REMOVAL OF UTERUS VAGINALLY

Trial Vaginal Route: Wherein 'TRIAL' is not for hysterectomy but the vaginal route is under Trial for extra uterine pathology, i.e. adnexal mass needing VH plus salpingo-oophorectomy.

We sincerely hope and look forward to colleagues to go beyond routine vaginal hysterectomy and offer advantages of vaginal route as well as keeping abdomen intact. Plentiful material will surely guide and inspire to put it into action.

What is Less Invasive?

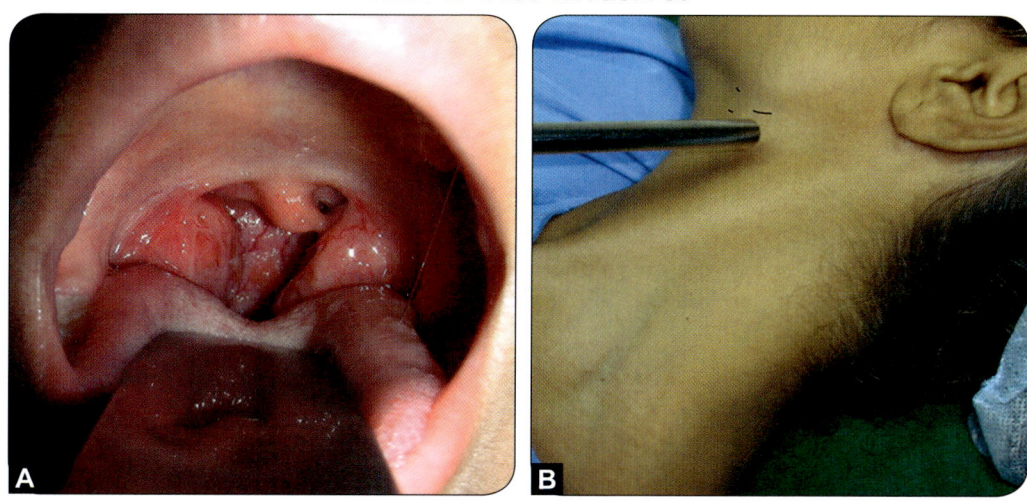

Figs. 1A and B: (A) Tonsils are seen and can be easily removed from the natural orifice just as the uterus can be seen and removed vaginally. This is less invasive than Fig.1B; (B) tonsils are removed via submandibular laparoscopy just as the uterus can be accessed for removal abdominally by laparoscope [Best Practice & Research – Clinical Obstetrics & Gynaecology. Edited by Prof. S. Arulkumaran, 2011;25(2):115-32.

Uterocervical Broad Ligament Space

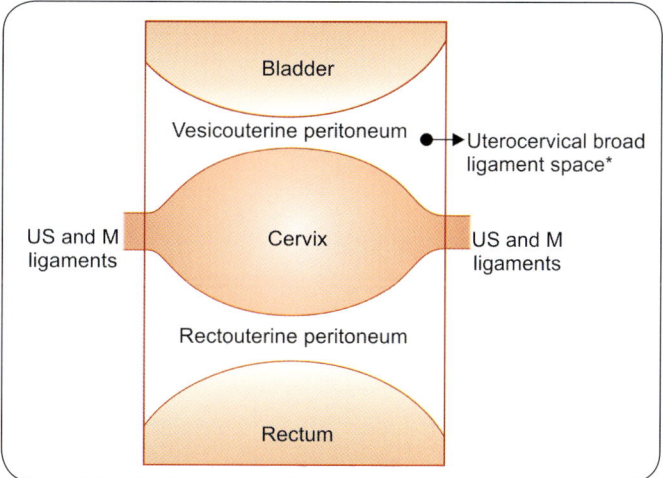

Fig. 2: Space between bladder and cervix or cervicouterine surface, which is much more under lateral one-fifth of bladder when compared with central three-fifths of bladder [Sheth SS. Access to vesicouterine and rectouterine pouches. In: Vaginal Hysterectomy, 2nd edition. New Delhi, India: Jaypee Brothers Medical Publishers (P) Ltd; 2014; pp. 31-50.].

---

*Sheth's uterocervical broad ligament space.

Same Longitudinal Dimension with Different Other Dimensions

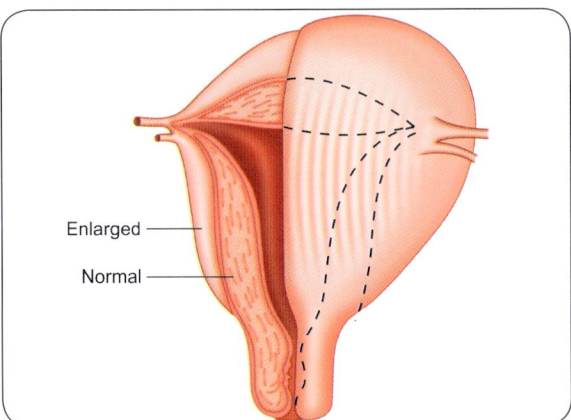

Fig. 3: Disproportionate multidimensional increase in uterine size (in AP and transverse dimensions compared with longitudinal) [Sheth SS. Newer Perspectives. Vaginal Hysterectomy, 2nd edition. New Delhi, India: Jaypee Brothers Medical Publishers (P) Ltd; 2014. pp. 225-234].

Start of Debulking

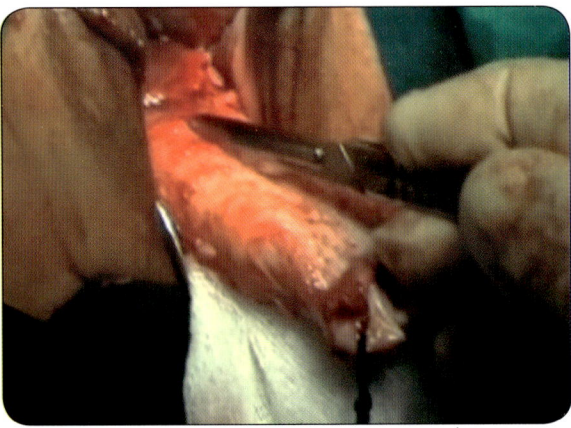

Fig. 4: Cervical bisection opens the passage for debulking.

Well Bisected Cervix and Part of Uterus for Debulking

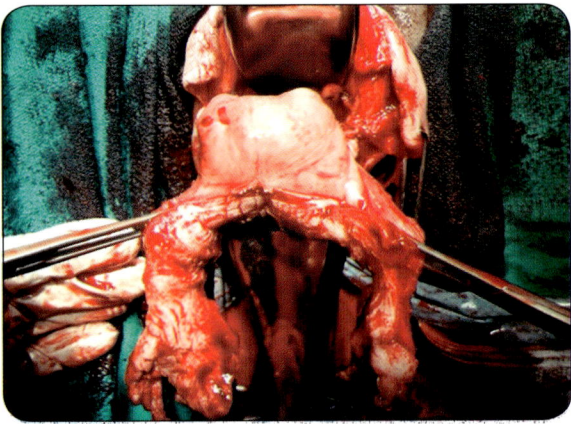

Fig. 5: Bisection of uterus [Goel N, Rajaram S, Jain S, Singh S. Trial vaginal hysterectomy and trial vaginal route. In: Sheth SS (Ed). Vaginal Hysterectomy, 2nd edition. New Delhi, India: Jaypee Brothers Medical Publishers (P) Ltd; 2014; pp. 116-122.

Debulking: Uterine Myoma Getting Enucleated

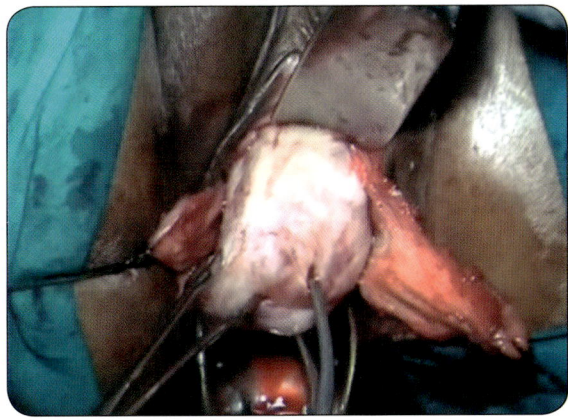

Fig. 6: Fibroid getting enucleated after cervical bisection.

Uterus Freed on Right with Left Ovarian Cyst

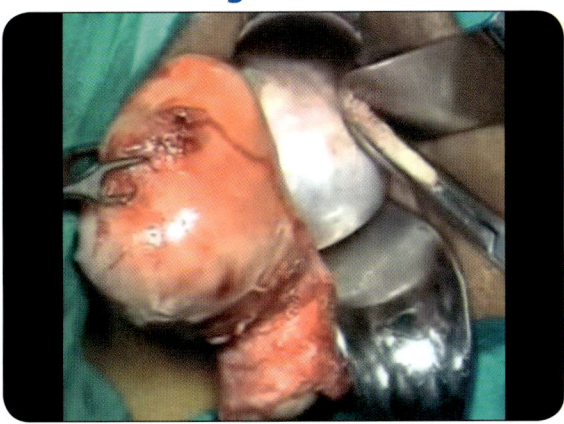

Fig. 7: Left ovarian tumor. All contralateral connections are severed to free the uterus for traction and perform salpingo-oophorectomy.

Ovarian Clamp for Clamping Infundibulopelvic Ligament

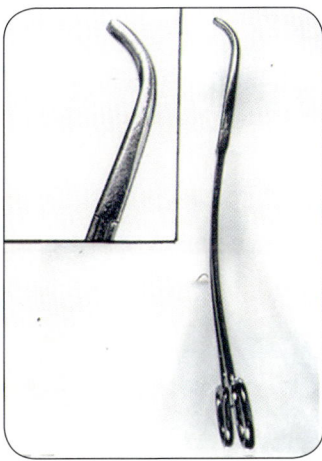

Fig. 8: Specially designed ovarian or Sheth adnexa clamp (Cooper Surgical, USA) [Br J Obstet & Gynecol, 1991;98:662-6.

Shirish S Sheth
Carl W Zimmerman
Seth Finkelstein

VAGINAL ROUTE IN GYNECOLOGY FOR HYSTERECTOMY WITHOUT ABDOMINAL ACCESS

INDICATIONS

Common Indications

Uterovaginal prolapse, abnormal uterine bleeding, uterine fibroids, adenomyosis, myomatous polyp, premalignant cervix and endometriosis. For some, good old 'Dysfunctional uterine bleeding'.

Uncommon Indications

- Vaginal hysterectomy (VH) with adnexectomy for benign pathology.
- VH for the management of menstruation in mentally compromised with intact hymen.
- VH for endometrial cancer.
- VH for cervical intraepithelial neoplasia or CIN III (Carcinoma-in-situ of cervix).
- VH for carcinoma cervix stage IA_1 (Invasion not more than 3 mm).
- VH with broad ligament myomectomy.
- Subtotal vaginal hysterectomy.
- Laparoscopic cholecystectomy and vaginal hysterectomy: A least invasive approach.
- Selectively, contraindicated conditions.

VAGINAL HYSTERECTOMY WITH ADNEXECTOMY FOR BENIGN PATHOLOGY WITHOUT LAPAROSCOPIC ASSISTANCE

For ovarian dermoid or such benign cyst, entire procedure of salpingo-oophorectomy can be achieved at vaginal hysterectomy, with adequate space for the operative procedure. For adnexal pathology, one does not have to change the route for hysterectomy from vaginal to abdominal for laparoscopic or opening of the abdomen. One can keep the abdomen intact.

Quite often, a cyst excised laparoscopically is removed through a posterior colpotomy. Then why not totally via vaginal route without laparoscope or abdominal cuts? The size of an ovarian cyst is not by itself a limiting factor, as the cyst can usually be aspirated and then excised. For the benign adnexal mass, operator will feel satisfied with adnexectomy at vaginal hysterectomy.[1-7]

VAGINAL HYSTERECTOMY FOR THE MANAGEMENT OF MENSTRUATION IN MENTALLY COMPROMISED

Most gynecologists are reluctant to attempt a vaginal hysterectomy because patient is a nullipara. Mentally compromised are not only nulliparous but additionally with intact hymen. Hysterectomy is mainly needed for menstrual hygiene and have performed vaginal hysterectomy in more than 120 such women and spared them from abdominal or laparoscopic hysterectomy.

Such hysterectomy can easily inspire to perform vaginal hysterectomy in nulliparous women.[7-11]

VAGINAL HYSTERECTOMY FOR ENDOMETRIAL CANCER

Vaginal hysterectomy has a definite place in the therapeutic armamentarium of the gynecology-oncologists for select women with endometrial cancer.

Author strongly recommends VH for postmenopausal bleeders with abnormal endometrial thickness and as such needing hysterectomy and also for those diagnosed endometrial cancer after hysteroscopy plus dilatation and curettage.

Vaginally removed uterus will be ideal for the frozen HP study and further management. It can spare from hysteroscopy plus dilatation and curettage (D&C) and many from more invasive abdominal access for hysterectomy. Comparatively, VH with bilateral salpingo-oophorectomy (BSO) is the least invasive surgery for the 'select' malignant and invasive condition.[7,12-14]

VAGINAL HYSTERECTOMY FOR CERVICAL INTRAEPITHELIAL NEOPLASIA (CIN) III (CARCINOMA-IN-SITU OF CERVIX)

If woman needs hysterectomy for CIN III, it will not be scientific to perform laparoscopically or by laparotomy. If not contraindicated, it should be the least invasive 'vaginal hysterectomy', preferably, with cuff of vagina.[13]

VAGINAL HYSTERECTOMY FOR CARCINOMA CERVIX STAGE IA$_1$ (INVASION NOT MORE THAN 3 MM)

It is exceedingly difficult to get a case of cancer cervix which is stage IA$_1$ in developing countries. One has to be very sure that invasion is not more. May be, preferably for a high-risk woman for surgery and pre and postoperative paraffin histopathology done with extra care.[7,15]

VAGINAL HYSTERECTOMY WITH BROAD LIGAMENT MYOMECTOMY WITHOUT LAPAROSCOPIC ASSISTANCE

Removal of a broad ligament fibroid vaginally at vaginal hysterectomy performed for a benign indication easily spares the patient from laparotomy or laparoscopic-assisted VH. The vaginal route does permit the enucleation of a broad ligament fibroid at VH without laparoscopic assistance.

This is particularly recommended to all vaginal surgeons performing a vaginal hysterectomy for large-sized uteri with salpingo-oophorectomy either prophylactic or for benign adnexal pathology at VH. Author has done more than 25 vaginal hysterectomies with concomitant broad ligament myomectomy without laparoscopic assistance.[5,7,16,17]

SUBTOTAL VAGINAL HYSTERECTOMY

Uncommonly, cervix is left behind. This is particularly when woman wants to preserve it and she is also keen to keep abdomen intact for the required hysterectomy, i.e. wants vaginal hysterectomy.

Subtotal vaginal hysterectomy needs extra care and expertise and may not be of choice for many gyencologists. However, it can certainly be done though not easy like total vaginal hysterectomy or abdominal subtotal hysterectomy in the same woman. In fact, extracts bit extra for the 'Topsy Turvy' from the operator.[7,18]

LAPAROSCOPIC CHOLECYSTECTOMY AND VAGINAL HYSTERECTOMY: A LEAST INVASIVE APPROACH

The surgeon and gynecologist can judiciously combine these two major operations in a single operative session, providing maximum benefits to their patients.

Thus, laparoscopic cholecystectomy combined with vaginal hysterectomy with or without salpingo-oophorectomy can be considered as the least invasive and with minimal access technique. This is advantageous in many ways.

The surgeon performing cholecystectomy should always exclude a gynecologic pathologic condition by abdomino-pelvic sonography, and vice-versa.

Similarly, VH can combine itself with several other surgeries like laparoscopic appendicectomy or hernia repair etc.[7,19-23]

SELECTIVELY, CONTRAINDICATED CONDITIONS

Contraindicated cases for vague and/or varied but genuine reasons, e.g. classical examples are twisted ovarian cyst, large cervical fibroid and ectopic pregnancy (needing hysterectomy).

REFERENCES

1. Yuen PM, Yu KM, Yip SK, Lau WC, Rogers MS, Chang A. A randomized prospective study of laparoscopy and laparotomy in the management of benign ovarian masses. Am J Obstet Gynecol. 1997;177(1):109-14.
2. Reich H, Foreword. In: Mettler l. (Ed.). Manual of New Hysterectomy Techniques. Jaypee Br.Med. Publishers (P) Ltd.. New Delhi; India: 2007;pp. xi-xii.
3. Pardi G, Carminati R, Ferrori MM, et al. Laparoscopically assisted vaginal removal of ovarian dermoid cysts. J Obstet Gynecol 1995; 85: 129-132.
4. Sheth SS. Adnexectomy for benign pathology at vaginal hysterectomy without laparoscopic assistance. Br. J Obstet Gynecol 2002; 109:1401-1405.
5. Sheth SS. Adnexal Pathology at vaginal hysterectomy. In: Sheth SS (Ed). Vaginal Hysterectomy, Second edition. New Delhi, India: Jaypee Brothers Medical Publishers (P) Ltd; 2014; pp 150-162.
6. Teng FY, Muzsnai D, Perez R, Mazdisnian F, Ross A, Sayre JW. A comparative study of laparoscopy and colpotomy for the removal of ovarian dermoid cysts. Obstet Gynecol. 1996;87(6):1009-13.
7. Sheth SS, Paghdiwalla KP, Hajari AR, Vaginal route: A gynaecological route for much more than hysterectomy. Best Practice & Research – Clinical Obstetrics & Gynaecology. Edited by Prof. S.Arulkumaran,Vol.25 (2):2011: 115-132.
8. Kaunitz AM, Thompson RJ, Kaunitz KK. Mental retardation: a controversial indication for hysterectomy. Obstet Gynecol. 1986;68(3):436-8.
9. Wheeless CR. Abdominal hysterectomy for surgical sterilization in the mentally retarded: a review of parental opinion. Am J Obstet Gynecol. 1975;122(7):872-5.
10. Sheth SS. The Nulliparous patient. In: Sheth SS (Ed). Vaginal Hysterectomy, Second edition. New Delhi, India: Jaypee Brothers Medical Publishers (P) Ltd; 2014. pp 63-71.
11. Sheth S, Malpani A. Vaginal hysterectomy for the management of menstruation in mentally retarded women. Int. J Gynecol Obstet 1991; 35: 319-321.
12. Zanagnolo V, Magrina JF. Vaginal hysterectomy for carcinoma of the endometrium. In: Sheth SS (Ed) Vaginal Hysterectomy, Second edition. New Delhi, India: Jaypee Brothers Medical Publishers (P) Ltd; 2014; pp 216-224.
13. Sheth SS. Vaginal or abdominal hysterectomy. In: Sheth SS (Ed). Vaginal Hysterectomy, Second edition. New Delhi, India: Jaypee Brothers Medical Publishers (P) Ltd; 2014; pp 273-293.
14. Zanagnolo V, Magrina JF. Carcinoma of the endometrium treated only by vaginal route. Best Practice & Research – Clinical Obstetrics & Gynaecology. Edited by Prof. S.Arulkumaran. Vol.25 (2):2011: 239-245.
15. Chi DS, Abu-Rustum NR, Plante M, Roy M. Cancer of the cervix. In: Rock JA, Jones HW, eds. Telinde's Operative Gynecology, 10th edn (Vol.2). Philadelphia: Lippincott Williams & Wilkins; 2008, pp 1227-1290.
16. Macleod D, Howkins J (Eds.). Hysterectomy for cervical and broad ligament myoma. Bonney's Gynaecological Sursgery, 7th Ed. London: William Clowes and Sons, Ltd., 1964; 253.
17. Sheth SS. Broad ligament myomectomy at vaginal hysterectomy without laparoscopic assistance. J Gynecol Surg 2007; 23: 133-141.
18. Magos A, Miskry T. Subtotal vaginal hysterectomy. In: Sheth SS (Ed) Vaginal Hysterectomy, Second edition. New Delhi, India: Jaypee Brothers Medical Publishers (P) Ltd; 2014; pp 163-171.
19. Pratt JH, O'Leary JA, Symmonds RE. Combined hysterectomy and cholecystectomy: A sudy of 95 cases. Mayo Clin Proc 1967; 42: 529.
20. Downs SH, Black NA, Devlin HB, Royston CMS, Russell RCG. Systematic review of the effectiveness and safety of laparoscopic cholecystectomy. Ann R Coll Surg Eng 1996; 78: 243.
21. Sheth SS, Bhansali SK, Goyal MV. Cholecystectomy and hysterectomy: A least invasive approach. J Gynecol Surg 1997; 13: 181-185
22. Bhansali SK, Sheth SS. Associated non-gynecological surgery. In: Sheth SS, Studd JWW, (eds). Vaginal Hysterectomy. London: Martin Dunitz Ltd., 2002, pp 237-242.
23. Udwadia TE, Sheth SS. Associated nongynecological surgery. In: Sheth SS (Ed). Vaginal Hysterectomy, Second edition. New Delhi, India: Jaypee Brothers Medical Publishers (P) Ltd; 2014; pp243-247.

Section 1: VAGINAL HYSTERECTOMY WITH UTERINE DEBULKING

> *"If you give a man more than he can do*
> *He will do it.*
> *If you only give him what he can do*
> *He will do nothing."*
>
> —R Kipling

CASES

Dr Shirish S Sheth

Introduction
Case 1: Vaginal Hysterectomy (VH) with Uterine Debulking
Case 2: Vaginal Hysterectomy (VH) with Uterine Debulking Plus Bilateral Salpingo-oophorectomy (BSO) (CA125: 516)
Case 3: Vaginal Hysterectomy with Uterine Debulking Plus Ovarian Cystectomy
Case 4: Vaginal Hysterectomy with Massive Uterine Debulking Plus Bilateral Salpingo-oophorectomy (Right Hydrosalpinx)
Case 5: Vaginal Hysterectomy with Debulking Plus Bilateral Salpingo-oophorectomy with H/O Two Caesarean Sections
Case 6: Vaginal Hysterectomy with Uterine Debulking Plus Bilateral Salpingo-oophorectomy and Laparoscopic Cholecystectomy

Dr Seth Finkelstein

Case 7: Nullipara: Large Debulking and Adnexectomy
Case 8: Nullipara and Obese: Debulking with Bilateral Salpingectomy
Case 9: Massive Debulking of Kilogram Uterus with Bilateral Salpingectomy-1
Case 10: Massive Debulking of Kilogram Uterus with Bilateral Salpingectomy-2
Case 11: Debulking of Large Adenomyoma, Bilateral Salpingectomy-1
Case 12: Debulking of Large Adenomyoma, Bilateral Salpingectomy-2
Case 13: Large Debulking with Bilateral Salpingectomy for Recurrent Postmenopause Bleeding
Case 14: Early Debulking with the Aid of Vasopressin

INTRODUCTION

Uterine debulking: This can get more interesting by any additional factor to deal with, such as a history of caesarean section or an associated adnexal pathology, e.g. VH for a large uterus with history of (H/O) caesarean section(s) in the past, or VH for a large uterus with benign ovarian cyst.

DEBULKING

- If uterine size is the only disturbing or distressing factor to undertake VH, the uterus upto reachable size can be easily debulked and help the operator to routinely undertake the technique and perform VH. However, debulking has its limit and the limit varies with uterine size as well as the skill of the operator. The definition of such a limit or reach depends on the operator's God given skill and courage and rises with increasing experience and success and failures. If one operates beyond one's limit, it invites complications. In the best interests of patients let favorable literature or hospitals and/or colleague's routine not dissuade or stop one from performing possible debulking without difficulty.
- Debulking is usually required for a uterine size bigger than 10–12 weeks or uterine volume more than approximately 200–250 cm³. It is almost mandatory to secure both uterine vessels before undertaking debulking. If done earlier, it could predispose to excessive bleeding. Uncommonly, an obstructing cervical fibroid may necessitate enucleation to facilitate reaching the uterine vessels. Intraoperatively, debulking will permit an access which is further or higher. Debulking is considered and comes into action only when uterine lateral connections are no more available to be severed and upper border of the uterus, i.e. fundus is distally placed and not felt from either anterior or posterior.[1]
- The method to debulk will depend on the uterine size, pathology behind the increased size and pathological site. Enucleation of a fibroid (myoma), morcellation of adenomyotic uterine walls and/or fibroid are the most common methods used. To debulk a uterine fibroid is easier than debulking an adenomyotic uterus. Usually both require cervical bisection from the external os to higher-up to access the site for debulking. Occasionally enucleation of the fibroid is possible without bisecting the cervix, just by incising the serosa of the bulging uterine wall.[1,2]
- In practice, it is wise not to take a decision to debulk only on the basis of good old fundal height of the uterus but also strongly consider the uterine volume. In fact, the author depends much more on the uterine volume than on the uterine size in weeks which is judged only from the fundal height.[3]
- CA125: Raised levels are not uncommon with benign gynecological pathology. The gynecologist should not lose his or her patient or case to an oncologist colleague just because of "raised CA125". Oncology surgeons may not be knowledgeable of benign gynecological conditions raising CA125 or may prefer to believe "raised CA125 means more likely to be malignancy". It is important to know this well.[4]
- A debulkable uterus should not contraindicate the vaginal route for the hysterectomy but let "debulking" become an integral part or step of VH for an enlarged uterus, and provide to both the doctor and patient reassurance of keeping away an abdominal access and greater invasion.

METHOD (TECHNIQUE)

For easy access to the fibroid (myoma) and/or to the inner uterine wall, cervical bisection is carried out from the external os to as high as possible and the accessible uterine walls are excised from within, keeping the uterine serosa intact. This may give sufficient ascent to reach the lower end of the fibroid(s) for easy enucleation. Once the tail of the fibroid is reached, the fibroid is secured, as the rest of the fibroid can be accessed without difficulty, i.e. separation of the fibroid from the surrounding uterine wall, followed by morcellation and/or enucleation. Usually the field is dry as debulking is done only after the uterine vessels are secured.[1]

A posterior wall fibroid is more accessible and therefore easier to tackle than an anterior wall fibroid. Similarly an anterior one is less difficult to deal with than a fundal fibroid. Larger the uterus the more distal is the fundal fibroid to access and worse to handle.

An attempt to reach the posterior wall is made by cutting the posterior uterine wall further upwards, and/or by debulking the uterine walls from inside on both sides, keeping the serosa intact. This is likely to give an access to more fibroids for morcellation and enucleation or access to a large posterior wall fibroid for morcellation and enucleation. The freed higher lateral connections are severed to facilitate further debulking.[1]

Continuation of the entire process helps in reaching higher and higher to the largest anterior wall or fundal fibroid, which is separated alround as far as possible and comfortably morcellated to advance to a size that can be enucleated. When this proves inadequate, one turns to the available anterior and/or posterior uterine walls for further bisection and continues morcellation and/or enucleation. This debulking makes more lateral uterine connections available for severance to avoid tear of small vessels. With an enlarged pathological uterus there is increased vascularity and therefore, it is essential to secure the small blood vessels laterally. Myoma screw can be used if required or if one is used to it. Dissection is almost avascular or with minimal oozing which can be cauterized.

When the uterine enlargement is selectively on the right or left side because of the location of a large fibroid, intraoperatively during debulking, the contralateral tube and ovary often pop out or come out from the pouch of Douglas or nearby. They pop out despite some of the lateral connections. This is being intact, needs to be secured. As a consequence of the traction applied to the uterus to the opposite side, tear of the popping tube and mesosalpinx near proximal cornual end is likely. Therefore, it is worth applying a clamp to that upper pedicle and excise the tube and utero-ovarian ligament from the uterus. This will prevent cornual tear and slippage of the pedicle laterally resulting in hemorrhage necessitating laparoscopy and/or laparotomy. Usually uterus is much larger on the contralateral side with the cornual area distally placed.

Once it appears that it will be possible to bring out the fundus from the posterior or even the anterior and this is done by traction on the residual part of the sizeable fibroid or uterine wall aided by suprapubic pressure. Alternatively, if possible, the author strongly recommends to pass a finger from the space near the cornual area from the posterior or behind to the anterior and bring it out in front, thus isolating the upper pedicle (tube and utero-ovarian ligament with or without round ligament) for clamping and excision. If thin peritoneum is seen covering the finger, it should be cut for the finger to penetrate and come out in the front.[5] Excision of the pedicle may be done in two parts, by clamping from above and by another overlapping clamp from below upwards so as to cover the entire tissues. This frees the uterus from all the lateral connections on one side as well as provides space to put a bladder retractor. The finger from the pouch of Douglas to the front and/or from the front to behind the fundus ascertains absence of adhesions. With the uterus free on one side, access and excision of the contralateral upper pedicle with or without salpingo-oophorectomy becomes easier to complete the hysterectomy.

When the uterus is unduly large—more than 16–18 weeks size, reaching even the bottom or tail of a large fibroid, particularly fundal or anterior wall fibroid is very satisfying. It will facilitate to separate the fibroid all-round and morcellate and/or enucleate as required to debulk the uterus. When a previously diagnosed fibroid is not a fibroid but adenomyoma or adenomyotic uterine wall, progressive morcellation will help to debulk and deliver the uterus. Morcellation is often heavy. One needs to be 100% sure that the entire debulking is well within the serosal layer of the uterus.

If the finger cannot reach the bottom or tail of the fibroid but can feel only the uterine cavity and uterine walls, it demands bisecting the available uterine wall further, anteriorly and/or posteriorly to get an access to the fibroid from within the uterine cavity for debulking.

If even this does not permit the delivery of the uterine fundus or reach upper pedicle(s), the alternate is to bisect the remaining uterus till the fundus, if possible, and make two halves of the uterus. Then gently push one half with its intact upper pedicle distally inside, keeping the cervical portion easily accessible. A gauze pack is pushed in well beyond the pouch of Douglas with part of it hanging outside, to keep the bowels and omentum away. This makes the open field wider for access. Both ovaries and tubes are inspected. If normal and desired, they are preserved. They should always be inspected at every VH to confirm normalcy. Traction on the free half of the hemihysterectomized uterus helps to complete salpingo-oophorectomy if indicated followed by dealing similarly with the remaining half of the uterus with the upper pedicle which was earlier pushed inside, i.e. to complete the removal of contralateral hemihysterectomized uterus with or without salpingo-oophorectomy and thus complete total VH with or without bilateral salpingo-oophorectomy.[1,2] Cervical bisection does not per se debulk but opens the door and facilitates debulking. Total bisection from the cervix to the fundus does not remove any uterine substance but it provides space to reach higher and permits completion of the hysterectomy.

When total uterine bisection is not possible and the fundus is distally placed and all available lateral connections severed, it is frustrating for the gynecologist to give up and use a laparoscope or open the abdomen. However, perseverance and optimism may answer these issues. Further bisection of the anterior and/or posterior uterine wall and excision or chopping of the uterine wall from inside can provide the required access and lead to success.

When debulking fails and operator is stuck, laparoscopic surgery will solve and prevent an opening of the abdomen.

During surgery the author always uses a long gauze piece, half of it being pushed into the pouch of Douglas and higher to get soaked and keep the bowels and omentum away and the remaining dry half hangs outside the vulva. This provides total safety in not losing a mop or gauze piece inside the peritoneal cavity. The soaked gauze is immediately changed. When much more of packing or gauze is required, like at salpingo-oophorectomy at VH, roller gauze is used and adherence to the same principle of half or less hanging outside the vulva.

Since more than a decade, the author does not close the peritoneum.[6] Sometimes wonders at why he closed the peritoneum for so many years! The next step is to perform McCall's or its modification by approximating the utero-sacral ligaments after taking bites on the distal peritoneum covering the bowel. This is followed by anchoring of all four pedicles—two uterosacrals with Mackendrot's and two upper pedicles including round ligaments to the vault, even though the upper pedicle has hardly any strength to offer. It is not uncommon to resort to for anterior and/or posterior colporrhaphy, even though it is not large "cele", it is a good opportunity to concurrently perform and give the benefit of it to the patient. It is unfortunate that at a laparoscopic or abdominal hysterectomy, cysto-rectoceles and perineum are not looked for and often if present, they remain unattended even by the pelvic floor experts and/or lovers.

The patient is given liquid diet on the same evening. I prefer to go slow for a few hours. It is satisfying to discharge the patient after 24–36 hours, so as to reduce unnecessary queries to doctors and/or nurses by telephone calls. After 24 hours the self-retaining catheter is removed to allow the patient to pass urine on her own, have intestinal peristalsis and improve food intake. In other words, she is freely mobile, physiologically fit and can go home.

WHY NOT ABDOMINAL HYSTERECTOMY?

This is because VH is the least invasive and scientifically in the best interests of patients as long as it can be safely done. Uterine size can contraindicate hysterectomy via the vaginal route and therefore, the usual choice is to do laparoscopic hysterectomy or laparoscopically-assisted vaginal hysterectomy (LAVH) and when that is not possible, abdominal hysterectomy.

For a uterine size of less than 18 weeks size, abdominal hysterectomy is totally avoidable. In fact, it can be said to be contraindicated in the interests of the patient, as long as an alternative like laparoscopic technique is available and can be done. Factually, when vaginal and laparoscopic hysterectomy are not contraindicated, opening the abdomen and performing hysterectomy for a uterus less than 18–20 weeks size or uterine volume less than 500–600 cm^3 is unscientific, taking the patient for a "ride" and tantamounts to cheating. Institute for Health and Clinical Excellence guidelines, Royal College of Obstetricians and Gynaecologists (RCOG) 2011, states that the only real indication necessitating total abdominal hysterectomy is uterine size greater than about 18 weeks.[7] It further says that in United Kingdom (UK) 67% of hysterectomies are still being carried out by open surgery and women are not being offered the full range of available treatments and are being "short changed".[7]

WHY UNDERTAKE VAGINAL HYSTERECTOMY?

- It is in the best interests of suffering women
- Favorable findings for debulking the uterus
- Back up experience of debulking
- No other contraindication
- Zeal to avoid more invasive alternatives.

When debulking is contraindicated, VH is contraindicated for a uterine size of more than 12–14 weeks or volume greater than approximately 250–400 cm^3.

There should be no hesitation to utilize laparoscopic surgery in difficult cases and complete the hysterectomy and if necessary, laparotomy but avoid complications. Laparoscopic or laparotomy is indicated when:
- Unduly large uterus for debulking
- VH is not possible, i.e. "Trial VH" fails or is not worth undertaking
- No further access for completing VH
- Uncontrolled bleeding during VH.

MORCELLATION

Assessment of the risk of sarcomatous spread from the morcellation of a myoma or fibroid: Sarcomatous change is very uncommon. Rapid growth of uterine size and/or poor response to gonadotropin-releasing hormone (GnRH) in reduction of uterine size should arouse suspicion of this entity. If sarcoma is suspected, it is better to remove the intact uterus abdominally and send it for frozen section histopathology (HP) study. When in doubt, frozen HP study becomes mandatory. For sarcomatous spread resulting from morcellation of undiagnosed fibroid at VH, one must note that the vagina communicates freely with the peritoneal cavity only via the anterior and posterior pouches. During fibroid morcellation, anterior entry to the peritoneal cavity is blocked or protected by the bladder retractor and anterior uterine wall and posterior entry is protected by a self-retaining Auward's speculum plus a gauze pack besides the uterine wall. Additionally isolation plastic sheet in the pouch of Douglas and the surrounding area is totally protective. Peritoneal contents and large cavity are far away. Morcellation is done with knife and scissors well within the uterine serosal wall and chopped material freely comes out without the slightest chance to touch or reach intact tissues and the higher placed peritoneal cavity. Therefore, to apply the litigational aspects linked with laparoscopic morcellation, is stretching it a bit too far or an excuse to avoid the vaginal route. In fact, many fibroids can be enucleated without morcellation or with little morcellation. Hence there is a wide difference between laparoscopic morcellation done in the peritoneal cavity abdominally[8] and morcellation done vaginally with a well-protected pouch of Douglas as well as vesicouterine space, open to exterior. Not to forget that laparoscopic morcellation can result in parasitic myomas in 0.95% or less cases.[8] This is unlikely at VH as the small open surgical field is well protected.

In performing vaginal hysterectomy, the crux lies in separating the bladder to get an access to the vesicouterine peritoneum and anterior pouch or peritoneal cavity. Bladder separation will also facilitate bisecting the cervix upwards, as high as required. It is clear that if the bladder is unseparated, cervical bisection will get restricted and bladder and occasionally the ureter is at risk for trauma. Satisfactory bladder separation is a must before debulking. Bladder separation from laterally in women with a H/O caesarean section permits easy access to secure lateral ligamentous pedicles and uterine vessels, which is a "*must*" before uterine debulking.

Except for select cases with a cervical fibroid, debulking does not supercede bladder separation and uterine vessels excision. Larger uterine size per se does stretch the adhesions and if anything it may make bladder less adherent and more separable.

Prerequisites are:
- Bladder separation and securing uterine vessels.
- Opening the pouch of Douglas (accessing rectouterine peritoneum).

Once the bladder is well separated and vesicouterine peritoneum is reached/opened, debulking gets all the attention and needed expertise and H/O a caesarean section in the past loses its importance.

Minus side: Larger sized uterus can have:
- Increased vascularity. Therefore, infiltration of saline with adrenaline 1 in 200,000 to 300,000 and the anesthesiologist keeping an eye on blood pressure to maintain it around 110/70–80 mm Hg and not much higher so as to reduce oozing or bleeding
- Vesicouterine peritoneum is at a distance
- Anxiety and phobia of failure.

Cervical fibroid has an obstructive value but it should not obstruct the mindset of the operator.

DEBULKING

Objective is to debulk, reach close to the uterine fundus and complete the hysterectomy.
- Secure uterine vessels. This is a prerequisite before debulking starts
- Bisect cervix upwards to include the lower uterine portion
- Morcellate thick uterine walls from inside, keeping serosa intact
- Enucleate small myomas to reach higher and morcellate large myoma(s) so as to facilitate enucleation
- Available lateral uterine connections are secured to facilitate further bisection of uterus till one reaches the lower pole or tail of the large fibroid
- Intraoperatively, if tube and ovary are popping out, clamp them near the cornu and secure them to avoid tear/bleeding. "Popping" additionally help accessing that cornual area so as to make the uterus free on one side
- If required, bisect more and more of the uterine walls upwards and enucleate small fibroids to reach a large fibroid and if required, bisect entire uterus into two halves and deal with each half separately.

REFERENCES

1. Sheth SS. Rathi MR. Uterine fibroids. In: Sheth SS (Ed). Vaginal Hysterectomy, 2nd edition. New Delhi: Jaypee Brothers Medical Publishers (P) Ltd; 2014. pp. 72-89.
2. Pelosi MA II, Pelosi MA III. Uterine debulking at vaginal hysterectomy. In: Sheth SS (Ed). Vaginal Hysterectomy, 2nd edition. New Delhi: Jaypee Brothers Medical Publishers (P) Ltd; 2014. pp. 90-109.

3. Sheth SS, Shah NM. Preoperative sonographic estimation of uterine volume: an aid to determine the route of hysterectomy. J Gynecol Surg. 2002;18:13-22.
4. Sheth SS, Ray SS. Severe adenomyosis and CA125. J Obstet Gynecol. 2014;34:79-81.
5. Sheth SS. Vaginal hysterectomy in women with a history of 2 or more caesarean deliveries. Int J Gynecol Obstet. 2013;122:70-4.
6. Peritoneal closure. Royal College of Obstetricians and Gynaecologists (RCOG) Guideline No 15. London, UK: RCOG Press; 2002.
7. Barton-Smith P. Clinical practice: Modernising hysterectomy surgery–is robotics the answer? RCOG Member Mat. 2011;1(1):14-15.
8. Van der Meulen JF, Pijnenborg JM, Boomsma CM, et al. Parasitic myoma after laparoscopic morcellation: a systematic review of the literature. BJOG. 2016;123(1):69-75.

CASE 1: VAGINAL HYSTERECTOMY (VH) WITH UTERINE DEBULKING

Name: Mrs. X
Age: 40 years
Obstetric history: 1 FTND (Full Term Normal Delivery)
No H/O abdominopelvic surgery.
Not obese with no H/O hypertension or diabetes.
Clinically pelvic findings: Easily palpable abdominally, 16 weeks size nodular uterus with physiological or favorable descent of cervix to attempt vaginal hysterectomy. Fornices were clear except nodular fibroids were felt.

Sonography showed uterine volume 520 cm^3 with posterior wall fibroid 7 cm × 6.4 cm with other pelvic findings normal. (Normal uterine volume is 40–60 cm^3).[1]

Diagnosis: Uterine fibroids
Operation: Vaginal hysterectomy
What deters/dissuades: Contraindicated uterine size for VH.

Vaginal hysterectomy started as usual and uterine vessels were well secured. This was followed by bisection of cervix from external os to as high as on lower uterine portion (Fig. 1). Uterine thick walls were morcellated and small fibroids enucleated to reach higher. Freed lateral connections were well excised. This gave an access to the fibroid wall, which was morcellated and enucleated to reach higher (Fig. 2). However more debulking was needed through the uterine walls and extending the uterine bisection to as high a level as possible. This led to the tail of posterior wall fibroid to access further and morcellate and enucleate, deliver the debulked uterus and complete the hysterectomy.[2-10] Normal tubes and ovaries were preserved, hemostasis was checked and vaginal closure done.

Blood transfusion was not needed. Hospital stay was 2 days with an uneventful speedy postoperative recovery.

Histopathology examination showed uterus weighed 580 g, multiple uterine fibroids plus severe adenomyosis. No malignancy.

What inspired: Past experience.

LESSONS

- VH done without difficulty for uterus of 16+ weeks size. Posterior wall fibroid makes it easier.
- With experience, can be taken as "Trial VH" case.[11,12]

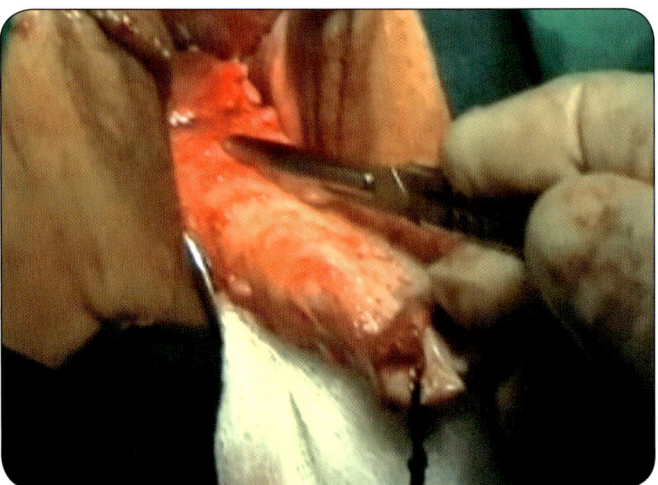

Fig. 1: After uterine vessels are secured, cervix is bisected to reach uterine cavity for the fibroid or its bulge.

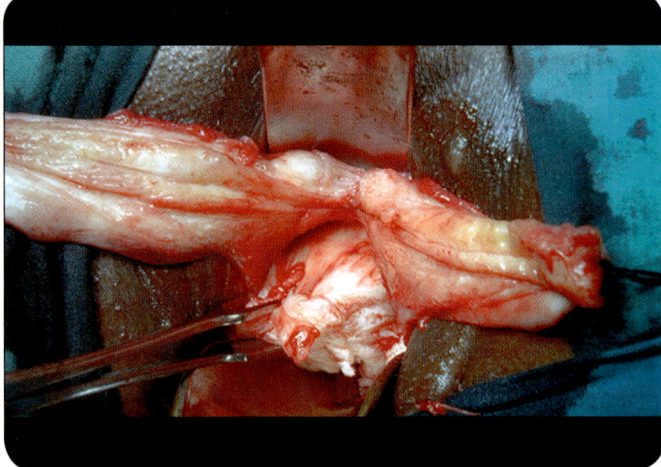

Fig. 2: Cervix bisected. Inner uterine walls morcellated to reach fibroid which is alround separated.

CASE 2: VAGINAL HYSTERECTOMY (VH) WITH UTERINE DEBULKING PLUS BILATERAL SALPINGO-OOPHORECTOMY (BSO) (CA125: 516)

Name: Mrs. X
Age: 50 years
Parity: 4 FTND
LD: 22 years back
Complains of (C/O): Heavy, painful menses with unbearable lower abdominal pain.

Not obese with no H/O hypertension or diabetes.

Clinically uterus 20 weeks size with favorable descent of cervix to attempt VH. Fornices were clear except a bulging uterus could be felt.

Uterus 11.8 cm × 8.5 cm × 13.8 cm volume 747 cm³. Adenomyotic without fibroids. Endometrial thickness 8 mm. Ovaries were normal. CA125 rose to 516.

Diagnosis: Large uterus with severe adenomyosis.[13,14]
Operation: VH with bilateral salpingo-oophorectomy. "Trial VH" case.[11,12]
What deters/dissuades VH: Large size uterus.

Vaginal hysterectomy done with required debulking after cervical bisection as high as possible.[4-6] Debulking was morcellation of thick adenomyotic uterine walls, with more and more of bisection of uterus and further morcellation (Fig. 1). Routine prophylactic bilateral salpingo-oophorectomy was performed as desired by the patient (Age: 50 years). Hemostasis was checked and vaginal closure done. Blood transfusion was not needed. Hospital stay was 2 days followed by an uneventful speedy recovery.

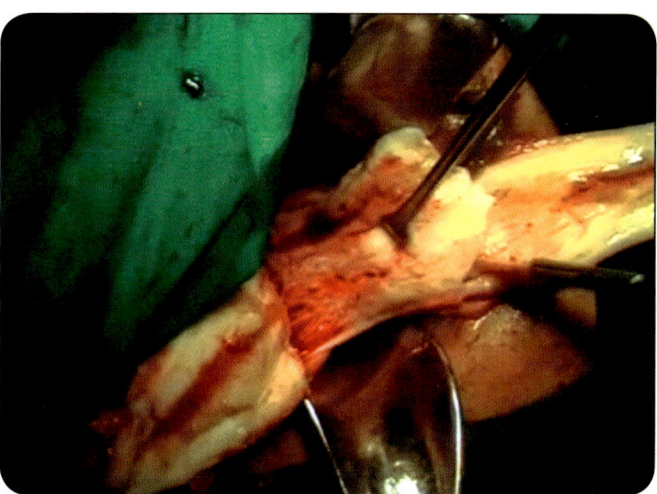

Fig. 1: Debulking of thick uterine walls. Bisected cervix—two halves seen well.

Histopathology showed uterus weighed 875 g with severe adenomyosis. Endometrium was normal with normal tubes and ovaries. No malignancy. About 6 weeks later CA125 returned to normal. The earlier reading was 516.[15]
What inspired: Uterine size and adenomyosis.

LESSONS

- Raised CA125 of 516 due to severe adenomyotic uterus. No malignancy
- 20 weeks size uterus debulked.

CASE 3: VAGINAL HYSTERECTOMY WITH UTERINE DEBULKING PLUS OVARIAN CYSTECTOMY

Name: Dr X
Age: 47 years
Parity: 2 FTND
LD: 12 years back
C/O: Heavy frequent menses. H/O hysteroscopy plus dilation and curettage (D&C) in 2013 with benign endometrium.

Not obese with no H/O hypertension or diabetes.

Clinically nodular uterus, 18 weeks size with favorable descent of cervix to attempt VH. Presence of cystic, tender mass in right fornix.

Sonography showed uterine volume was 525 cm^3 with right ovarian cyst of 2 cm × 2 cm with calcification and without solid area or internal echoes. Left adnexa normal.
Diagnosis: Uterine fibroids with adenomyosis plus right ovarian cyst.
Operation: VH with right ovarian cystectomy. "Trial VH" and "Trial vaginal route" case.[12]
What deters/dissuades VH: Size with adnexal mass.

VH started in usual manner. Uterus had severe adenomyosis plus leiomyomatous. Debulking was done after uterine vessels were secured by bisecting the cervix and lower anterior uterine wall, morcellating the uterine walls and fibroids and enucleating fibroids (Fig. 1). Thereafter hysterectomy was completed.[3-5,10,12,16,17]

Right ovary had unhealthy 2 × 2 cm calcified, hard area which was excised and sent for frozen HP study (Fig. 2). Frozen HP report showed right ovarian cystadenoma without malignancy. Raw area was sutured and right ovary was preserved as the patient was keen to preserve both her ovaries (Age: 47 years). Thus VH plus right ovarian cystectomy was done.[18,19] After checking hemostasis, vaginal closure was done. Blood transfusion was not needed. Hospital stay was 2 days. Postoperative was uneventful with speedy recovery.

Histopathology examination showed uterus weighed 643 g with severe adenomyosis and leiomyomatous and no malignancy. Ovarian cyst was benign cystadenoma. No malignancy.
What inspired: Past experience.

LESSON

- Benign mobile ovarian cyst for adnexectomy added flavor and not inhibition.

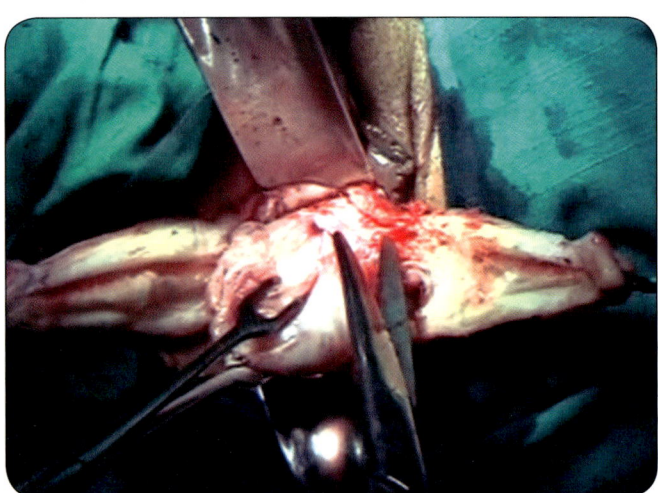

Fig. 1: Bisect cervix to reach and enucleate fibroid.

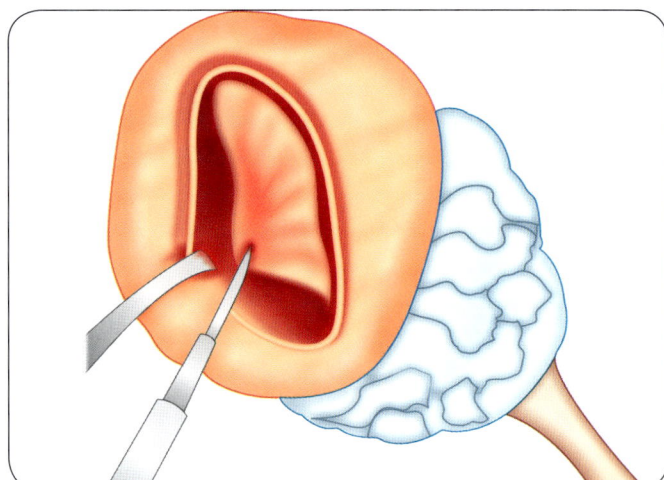

Fig. 2: Dissection of ovarian cyst wall.

CASE 4: VAGINAL HYSTERECTOMY WITH MASSIVE UTERINE DEBULKING PLUS BILATERAL SALPINGO-OOPHORECTOMY (RIGHT HYDROSALPINX)

Name: Mrs. X
Age: 49 Years
Parity: 2 FTND
LD: 12 years back
C/O: Heavy, frequent painful menses

Not obese but with hypertension with no H/O diabetes.

Uterus well felt abdominally 22–24 weeks size with physiological cervical descent. Large fibroids filling lateral and posterior fornix.

Sonography showed uterus 17 cm × 11.8 cm × 9.6 cm with endometrial thickness of 4 mm. Right fundal fibroid 7.5 cm × 7 cm and posterior wall fibroid 6.9 cm × 6.5 cm. Uterine volume 1,000 cm^3. Right tube showed hydrosalpinx (5 cm × 3 cm) with normal ovaries.

Diagnosis: Large uterus with fibroids.[20]

Operation: VH with bilateral salpingo-oophorectomy. "Trial VH" case.[11,12]

What deters/dissuades VH: Large uterine size.

Clinically and under anesthesia, cervical descent was favorable to attempt VH as "Trial VH" case (Figs. 1 and 2A and B). "Trial" because of uterine size. Uterine vessels were secured, the cervix bisected and debulking of uterine walls and small fibroids was done to reach the large posterior wall fibroid. This was carefully separated alround, morcellated and enucleated. Debulking of uterine adenomyotic walls by morcellation, enucleation of small fibroids continued, thus securing available lateral connections. Uterus was further bisected to debulk and gradually reach the tail of the fundal fibroid (Fig. 3) [myoma screw is not used by the author (Fig. 4)]. This was sufficiently morcellated to deliver the uterine fundus from posterior and secure

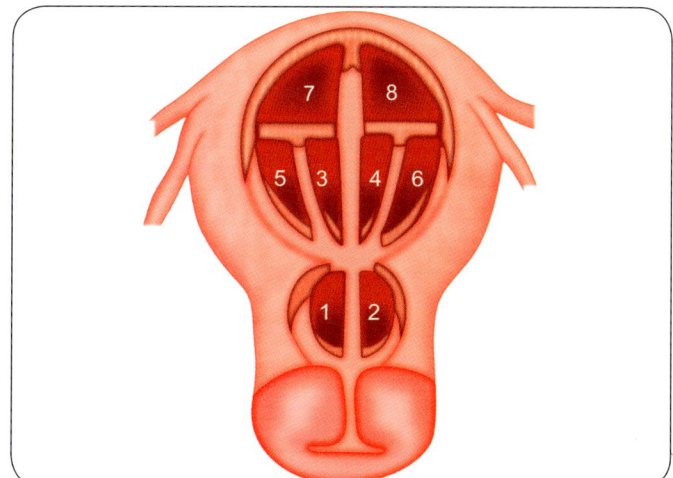

Fig. 1: Systematic anterior morcellation: Pryor's technique. With traction applied, wedges of the anterior uterine wall are removed in sequence, allowing the adnexal attachments to be pulled into view.[4] The figure shows good old morcellation technique for debulking.

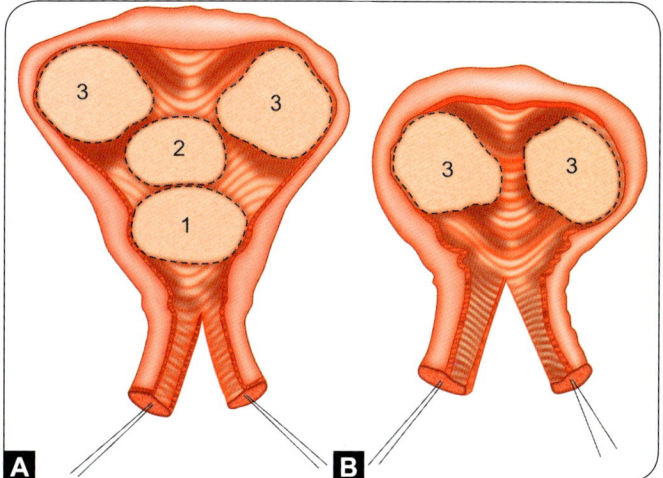

Figs. 2A and B: Debulking of the uterus of about 14 week's size, (A) by enucleation of the proximal central fibroid after bisection of the cervix followed; (B) enucleation of the distal fibroids.[5] Both the figures show located position of fibroids and technically how one approaches from below upwards for debulking.

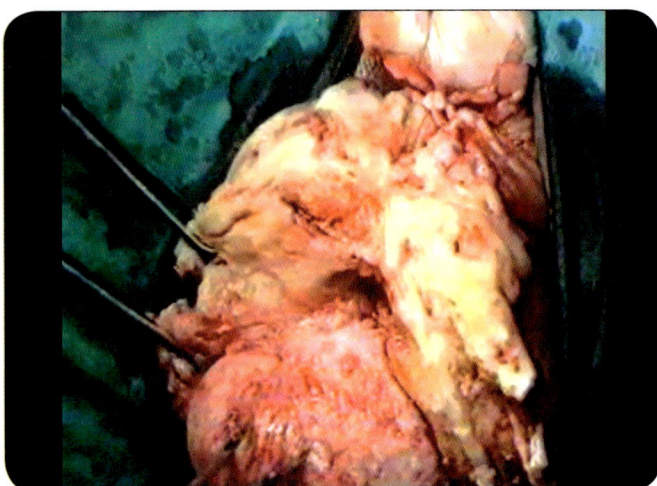

Fig. 3: Gratifying hysterectomy. Bisection, access and myomectomy.

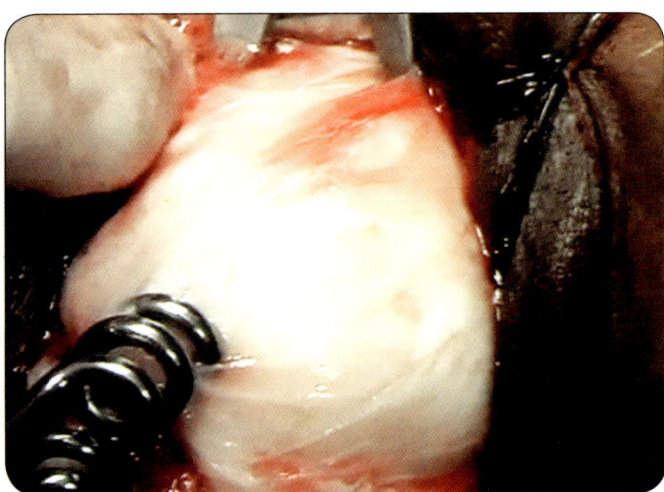

Fig. 4: Fundal fibroid, which is gripped with the screws, debulked and finally enucleated to deliver the fibroid and the entire uterus along with it.[5] Is not used in presented case.

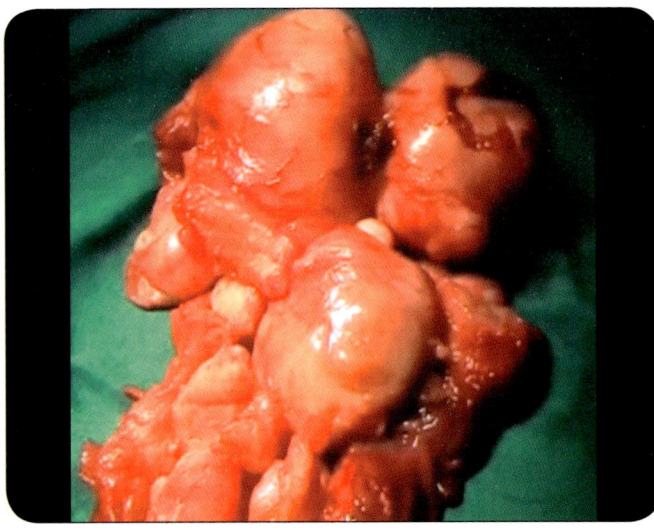

Fig. 5: Massive debulking as fibroids became easily accessible, one after other.

upper pedicles and complete hysterectomy with bilateral salpingo-oophorectomy[19,21-24] including hydrosalpinx. Patient was keen to have her ovaries removed. Hemostasis was checked and vaginal closure done (Fig. 5).

Blood transfusion was not needed. Hospital stay was 2 days with an uneventful speedy recovery.

Histopathology showed uterus weighed 1,148 g with multiple intact and morcellated fibroids. Both ovaries and left fallopian tube were normal with right tube showing hydrosalpinx and paratubal cyst. No evidence of malignancy.

What inspired: Past experience.

LESSON

- VH for 24+ week's size uterus should inspire many to undertake at least uterus less than 12 weeks size for VH.

CASE 5: VAGINAL HYSTERECTOMY WITH DEBULKING PLUS BILATERAL SALPINGO-OOPHORECTOMY WITH H/O TWO CAESAREAN SECTIONS

Name: Mrs. X
Age: 44 years
Parity: 2 FTCS
LD: 9 years back.
C/O: Heavy, frequent menses.
Last menstrual period (LMP): 10 days back.
The patient was not obese and did not have H/O hypertension or diabetes.

The uterus was 16 weeks size, mobile with fibroids. Cervical descent was favorable to attempt VH. Sonography showed an enlarged uterus of 560 cm^3 volume. Large posterior wall fibroid with normal tubes and ovaries.
Diagnosis: Uterine fibroids.
Operation: Vaginal hysterectomy with bilateral salpingo-oophorectomy.
What deters/dissuades VH: H/O 2 caesarean sections.

The anterior peritoneum was accessed via the uterocervical broad ligament space[25,26] (Fig. 1). The pouch of Douglas was accessed without difficulty as it was free followed by securing ligaments and uterine vessels. Bladder retractor was carefully and freely put between the cervicouterine surface and bladder. Cervix was then bisected as high as possible to get an access to lower pole of fibroid. This was followed by debulking the uterus by morcellation of the thick adenomyotic uterine walls and enucleation of the fibroids, particularly posterior wall fibroid. The lateral connections were secured on one side and further traction on the free uterus facilitated hysterectomy without difficulty. On naked eye examination, the endometrium was normal in the enlarged adenomyotic uterus with large sized and small fibroids. Hemostasis was checked and closure done. Blood transfusion was not needed. Hospital stay was 2 days followed by an uneventful, speedy recovery.

Histopathology study: Uterus weighed 630 g with severe adenomyosis plus large fibroid of 360 g and tubes and ovaries normal. No malignancy detected.
What inspired: Size of uterus with Caesarean sections in past.

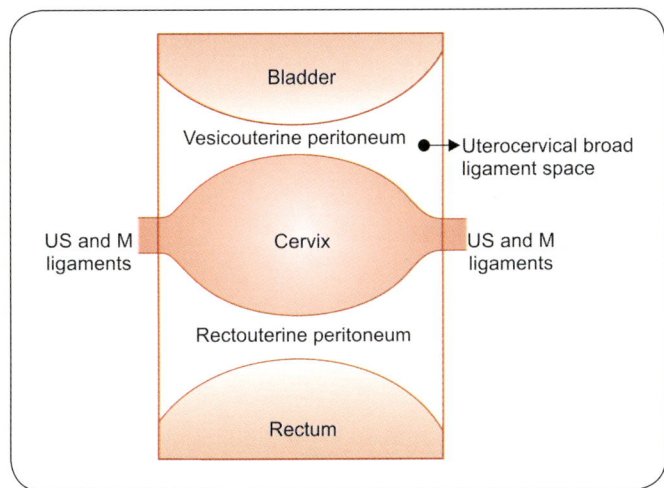

Fig. 1: Figure distinctly shows the space between bladder and cervix or cervicouterine surface, which is much more under lateral one fifth of bladder when compared with central three fifths of bladder.
[Sheth SS (Ed). Vaginal Hysterectomy, 2nd edition. New Delhi, India: Jaypee Brothers Medical Publishers (P) Ltd; 2014; pp. 31-50].

LESSON

- History of two Caesarean Sections added flavor.

CASE 6: VAGINAL HYSTERECTOMY WITH UTERINE DEBULKING PLUS BILATERAL SALPINGO-OOPHORECTOMY AND LAPAROSCOPIC CHOLECYSTECTOMY

Name: Mrs. X
Age: 43 years
Parity: 2 FTND
LD: 11 years back
C/O: Heavy painful menses

Not obese with no H/O hypertension or diabetes.

Uterus 18 weeks size, nodular with favorable cervical descent to attempt vaginal hysterectomy. Fornices were clear.

Sonography showed uterus 11.9 cm × 10.4 cm × 8.6 cm with uterine volume 465 cm^3 (Fig. 1). Additionally, she had symptomatic gallstones for which a surgeon strongly advised laparoscopic cholecystectomy[27] (Fig. 2).

Medically she was fit to undergo cholecystectomy as well as hysterectomy at the same session. This was discussed at length with the patient and her relatives and they were fully counseled.[28] She was also keen to have both surgeries done at the same time.

Diagnosis: Uterine fibroids plus gallstones.
Operation: Laparoscopic cholecystectomy followed by VH with bilateral salpingo-oophorectomy.
What deters/dissuades: If "Trial VH" fails.

Laparoscopic cholecystectomy was easily first performed by the surgeon and patient's position then changed to the lithotomy one.[28-31] VH was carefully done with required debulking after cervical bisection as high as possible[2,5,32] (Figs. 3A and B). Concomitant bilateral salpingo-oophorectomy at VH was done though she was 43 years old because of a H/O ovarian cancer in mother.[33]

Performing both major operations at the same time required only, one hospital admission, stay and one visit to the operation theater and anesthesia only once. Removing a large uterus of 500 g without abdominal access including different sites for laparoscopic hysterectomy than sites for the laparoscopic cholecystectomy. Hemostasis was checked and closure done. Blood transfusion was not needed. Hospital stay was 2 days. Postoperatively she made a speedy recovery.

Histopathology study showed uterus weighed 500 g with multiple leiomyoma, ovaries showed follicular cyst and tubes with paratubal cysts. No malignancy. Gallbladder showed acute and chronic calculous cholecystitis and no evidence of malignancy.

It was gratifying for the surgeon as well as the gynecologist and an inspiration for others.

What inspired: What was in the best interest of patient.

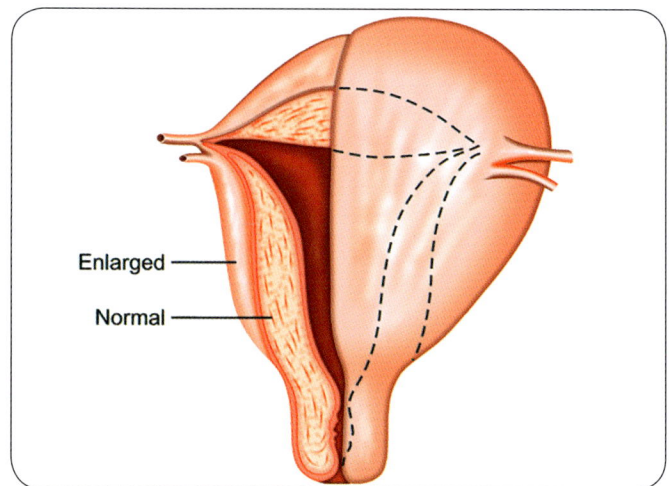

Fig. 1: Disproportionate multidimensional increase in uterine size (in AP and transverse dimensions compared with longitudinal).
Source: In: Sheth SS (Ed). Vaginal Hysterectomy, 2nd edition. New Delhi: Jaypee Brothers Medical Publishers (P) Ltd; 2014. pp. 225-34.

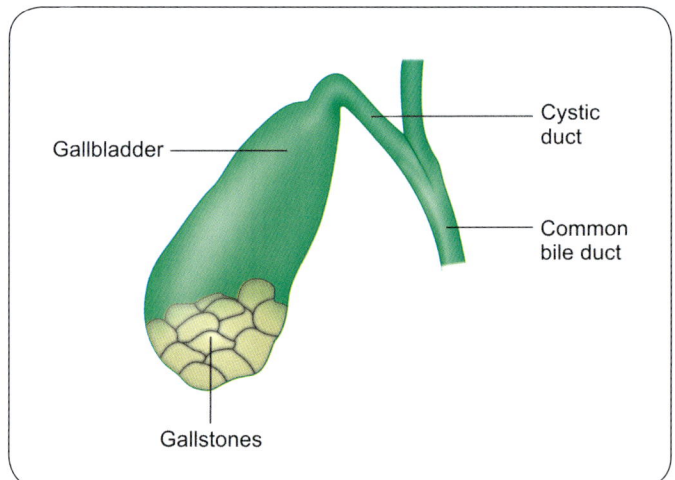

Fig. 2: Gallbladder with stones.

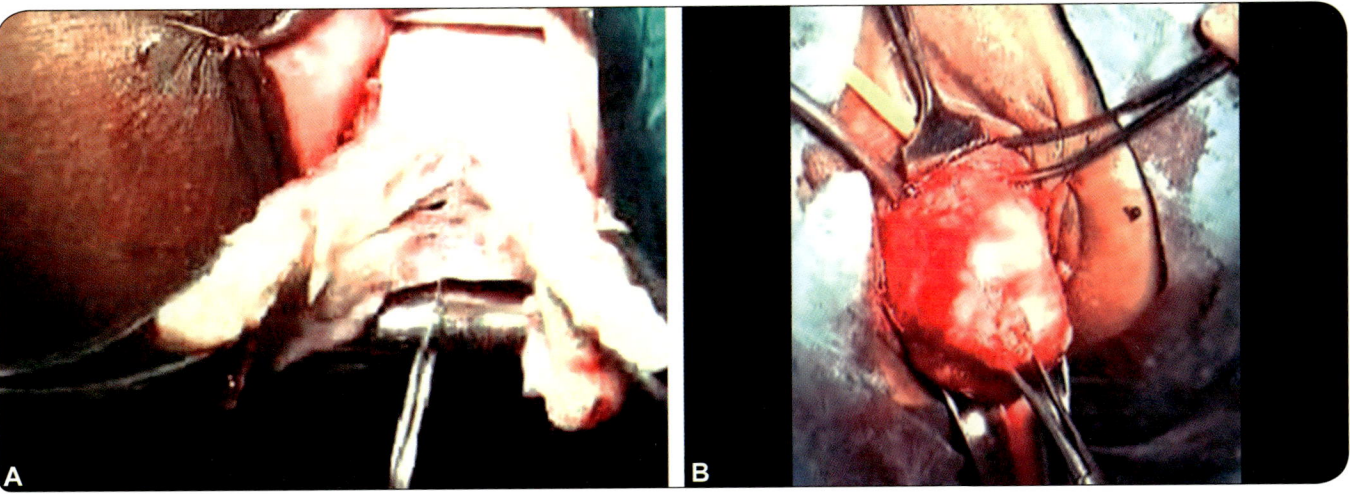

Figs. 3A and B: (A) Uterus is split vertically after ligating the uterine to reach the fibroid and (B) Fibroid is then enucleated to deliver it out.[5]

LESSONS

- Laparoscopic cholecystectomy gives an excellent opportunity to not only perform examination under anesthesia and if required, a good look through the laparoscope to evaluate the pelvic findings
- It is like killing two birds with one stone. Advantageous for patient and colleague.

REFERENCES

1. Sheth SS, Shah NM. Preoperative sonographic estimation of uterine volume: an aid to determine the route of hysterectomy. J Gynecol Surgery. 2002;18:13-22.
2. Pelosi MA III, Pelosi MA. The Pryor technique of uterine morcellation. Int J Gynecol Obstet. 1997;58:299-303.
3. Pelosi MA, Pelosi MA III. A comprehensive approach to morcellation of the large uterus. Contemp Obstet Gynecol. 1997;42:106-25.
4. Pelosi MA II, Pelosi MA III. Uterine debulking at vaginal hysterectomy. In: Sheth SS (Ed). Vaginal Hysterectomy, 2nd edition. New Delhi: Jaypee Brothers Medical Publishers (P) Ltd; 2014. pp. 90-109.
5. Sheth SS. Rathi MR. Uterine fibroids. In: Sheth SS (Ed). Vaginal Hysterectomy, 2nd edition. New Delhi: Jaypee Brothers Medical Publishers (P) Ltd; 2014. pp. 72-89.
6. Sheth SS. Vaginal hysterectomy or abdominal hysterectomy. In: Sheth SS, Sutton C (Eds), Menorrhagia. Oxford: ISIS Medical Media. 1999. pp. 213-37.
7. Lash AF. A method of reducing the size of the uterus in vaginal hysterectomy. Am J Obstet Gynecol. 1941;42:452.
8. Magos AL, Bournas N, Sinha R, et al. Vaginal hysterectomy for the large uterus. BJOG. 1996;103:246-51.
9. Nazah I, Robin F, Jais JP, et al. Comparison between bissection/morcellation and myometrial coring for reducing large uteri during vaginal hysterectomy or laparoscopically assisted vaginal hysterectomy: results of a randomized prospective study. Acta Obstet Gynecol Scand. 2003;82:1037-42.
10. American College of Obstetrics and Gynecology. Criteria for hysterectomy for leiomyomata. ACOG Tech. 1994;46:73-82.
11. Sheth SS. Vaginal hysterectomy. In: Studd J (Ed). Progress in Obstetrics and Gynecology, 10th edition. London: Churchill Livingstone; 1993. pp. 317-40.
12. Sheth SS, Paghdiwalla KP, Hajari AR. Vaginal route: A gynaecological route for much more than hysterectomy. Best Pract Res Clin Obstet Gynaecol. 2011;25(2):115-32.
13. Taran FA, Weaver AL, Coddington CC, et al. Characteristics indicating adenomyosis coexisting with leiomyomas: a case-control study. Hum Reprod. 2010;25:1177-82.
14. Taran FA, Wallwiener M, Kabashi D, et al. Clinical characteristics indicating adenomyosis at the time of hysterectomy: a retrospective study in 291 patients. Arch Gynecol Obstet. 2012;285:1571-76.
15. Sheth SS, Ray SS. Severe adenomyosis and CA125. J Obstet Gynecol. 2014;34:79-81.
16. Guvenal T, Ozsoy AZ. The availability of vaginal hysterectomy in benign gynecologic diseases: a prospective, nonrandomized trial. J Obstet Gynaecol Res. 2010;36:832-7.
17. Jones HW. Abdominal hysterectomy. In: Rock JA, Jones HW (Eds). Telinde's Operative Gynecology, Volume 1, 10th edition. Philadelphia: Lippincott Williams & Wilkins; 2008. pp. 727-43.
18. Sheth SS. The place of oophorectomy at vaginal hysterectomy: Br J Obstet Gynecol. 1991;98:662-6.
19. Sheth SS. Adnexectomy for benign pathology at vaginal hysterectomy without laparoscopic assistance. Br. J Obstet Gynecol. 2002;109:1401-5.
20. Sutton CJ. Treatment of large uterine fibroids. Br J Obstet Gynaecol. 1996;103(6):494-6.

21. Hoffman MS, DeCesare S, Calter C, et al. Abdominal hysterectomy vs transvaginal morcellation for the removal of enlarged uteri: Am J Obstet Gynecol. 1994;171:309-13.
22. Adanu RMK, Hammoud MM. Contemporary issues in women's health. Int J Obstet Gynecol. 2010;109:3-4.
23. Sheth SS. Adnexal pathology at vaginal hysterectomy? In: Sheth SS (Ed). Vaginal Hysterectomy, 2nd edition. New Delhi: Jaypee Brothers Medical Publishers (P) Ltd; 2014. pp. 150-62.
24. Sahen Y. Vaginal hysterectomy and oophorectomy in women with 12-20 weeks' size uterus. Acta Obstet Gynecol Scand. 2007;86:1359-69.
25. Sheth SS, Malpani AN. Vaginal hysterectomy following previous caesarean section. Int. J Gynecol Obstet. 1995;50:165-9.
26. Sheth SS. Vaginal Hysterectomy. Best Pract Res Clin Obstet Gynaecol. 2005;19(3):307-32.
27. Downs SH, Black NA, Devlin HB, et al. Systematic review of the effectiveness and safety of laparoscopic cholecystectomy. Ann R Coll Surg Eng. 1996;78:243.
28. Sheth SS, Bhansali SK, Goyal MV, et al. Cholecystectomy and hysterectomy: a least invasive approach. J Gynecol Surg. 1997;13:181-5.
29. Murray JM, Glistrap LC III, Massey FM. Cholecystectomy and abdominal hysterectomy. JAMA. 1980;244:2305.
30. Pratt JH, O'Leary JA, Symmonds RE. Combined hysterectomy and cholecystectomy: A study of 95 cases. Mayo Clin Proc. 1967;42:529.
31. Udwadia TE, Sheth SS. Associated nongynecological surgery. In: Sheth SS (Ed). Vaginal Hysterectomy, 2nd edition. New Delhi: Jaypee Brothers Medical Publishers (P) Ltd; 2014. pp. 243-7.
32. Pryor WR. The technique of vaginal hysterectomy. Am J Med. 1901;1:153-158.
33. The American College of Obstetricians and Gynecologists. Prophylactic oophorectomy (ACOG Practice Bulletin). Compendium of selected publication. Washington DC, USA: American College of Obstetricians and Gynecologists Women's Health Care Physicians. 2006. pp. 905-10.

CASE 7: NULLIPARA: LARGE DEBULKING AND ADNEXECTOMY

Name: Mrs. AMD
Age: 41 years
Parity: 0
Indication for surgery: Mass effect
Medical/surgical comorbidity: 0
Operative time: 4 hours 20 min (inclusive of cystoscopy and uterosacral colposuspension).
Hemoglobin (Hb) pre- and postoperative: 12 g/dL, 7 g/dL.
Recovery course: 2 units packed red blood cells (PRBC) transfused postoperative. Discharged postoperative day 1 (POD1) with Hb 9 g/dL. Minimal analgesic use, rapid return to baseline activity level.
Pathology report: Benign bilateral oviducts. Uterus 754 g, leiomyoma [add 10% to uterine weight, specimen sent directly in formalin to pathology. Gross weight directly in operation room (OR) would be 10–15% more].
Preoperative evaluation: Patient presented requesting hysterectomy. She strongly expressed that she had no interest in fertility. Her wishes were to restore life quality by permanently ending her longstanding daily suffering from uterine mass effect. Rapid return to work and activity was also of utmost importance to her and she thus was seeking a minimal invasive approach without any abdominal cuts if possible.

Pelvic exam revealed a readily accessible cervix and mobile large uterus.

Office TA and transvaginal (TV) ultrasound was performed with following findings:
- Estimated uterine weight 831 g
- Dominant large anterior fundal myoma, multiple additional smaller myomas
- Uterine dimensions of the lower segment 3 cm superior to cervix internal os were measured at 6 cm anteroposterior (AP) and 9 cm transverse. These findings strongly suggested uterine arteries would be accessible.

Magnetic resonance imaging (MRI) of pelvis was obtained to better delineate fibroid location and confirm that descent of lower segment dimensions were feasible for descent between ischial spines to allow for uterine artery access.

What deters/dissuades: Nulliparity with its associated limited vaginal space and limited uterine descent, all in setting of a very large uterus with most of its bulk anterior and thus obstructed from descent by pubic bone.

Surgery: Patient was consented as "Trial VH" with laparotomy conversion if needed. Ovarian preservation was agreed upon.

Sharp initial entry anteriorly into vesicouterine space (VUS) was direct and relatively straightforward. One must stay diligent to stay in correct plane along cervix to lower uterine segment. With large uterus, and especially one with anterior bulk, the angle of entry is more acute anterior toward pubic bone. Maintaining a traditional route of dissection will lead the surgeon subserosal on uterus and into bleeding.

Anterior dissection is taken only as apical as needed to safely divide uterosacral pedicles. The descent afforded by this step allows one to return to the anterior dissection and proceed apically sufficient to allow safe division of cardinal ligament pedicles and so on, with the surgeon continually reevaluating the anterior dissection below bladder after each step of operation.

After securing the uterine vessels, morcellation was very slowly but progressively accomplished with a combination of uterine bivalve and wedge resection. Individual myomas were enucleated as they became accessible. Impeding progress was the massive uterine volume and difficulty navigating the anterior bulk under pubis for safe morcellation under direct visualization. Upper pedicles on patient right were first to be accessed and divided. Right salpingectomy was performed. As morcellation progressed encouragingly with further descent of the uterine bulk, a sudden large hemorrhage ensued and it was noted that the descending pressure in the pelvis from traction on uterus caused partial avulsion of the right infundibulopelvic ligament. Securing the bleeding unfortunately required sacrificing the ovary on that side. The remainder of the surgery proceeded without further incident. Morcellation continued slowly until the left upper pedicles were reached and divided. The adnexa were readily accessible for removal of the oviduct, and the healthy normal left ovary was spared.

LESSONS

- Nulliparity, even in combination with large myomas, does not preclude VH
- Preoperative evaluation and planning are critical to success

- Appropriate preoperative counseling of patients is critical. Ultimately this was elective surgery. The patient was made to feel like a partner in the decision making process. This surgery was complicated by transfusion and unilateral oophorectomy, but patient remained extremely satisfied. She was fully informed about her surgical risks, and in the end her desires were met for a minimal invasive surgery, complete symptom relief, and return to normal activity
- Adnexa are readily accessible most cases
- Although uterine arteries have much greater blood flow, adnexal hemorrhages are often worse as they can take longer to identify and are more difficult to access.

CASE 8: NULLIPARA AND OBESE: DEBULKING WITH BILATERAL SALPINGECTOMY

Name: Mrs. TD
Age: 52 years
Parity: 0
Indication for surgery: Mass effect, menorrhagia.
Medical/surgical comorbidity: Body mass index (BMI) 32, hypothyroid.
Operative time: 3 hours 30 min (inclusive of cystoscopy and uterosacral colposuspension).
Hemoglobin pre- and postoperative: 11.8 g/dL, 8.4 g/dL.
Recovery course: Discharge day 1, minimal postoperative pain. Compression neuropathy of (R) peroneal nerve resulting in "foot drop" diagnosed postoperative. Patient required 6 months physical therapy, after which symptoms fully resolved without sequela.
Pathology report: Benign oviducts, uterus 500 g, leiomyoma (add 10% to uterine weight, specimen sent directly in formalin to pathology. Gross weight directly in OR would be 10–15% more).
Preoperative evaluation: Patient presented complaining of longstanding mass effect and increased menses during past year "so heavy I can't leave the house". Patient unemployed, but nonetheless effect on her life quality was profound. Pelvic exam revealed a 16-week mobile uterus and readily accessible cervix. Sonographic estimate of uterine weight was 435 g. Benign endometrial biopsy was obtained. Patient was offered "Trial VH" and counseled accordingly. Unsurprisingly, although work obligations were not a factor, the prospect of a minimal invasive vaginal operation as opposed to major abdominal operation was appealing to her.
What deters/dissuades: Nulliparity (limited space, descent), large uterine mass.

Surgery: VUS was sharply entered. Initial attempt to enter pouch of Douglas (POD) failed and posterior peritoneum retracted apically. Posterior entry had to be deferred until after division of cardinal ligament pedicles. Meanwhile, there was mild persistent bleeding in this retroperitoneal area.

Anterior dissection was revisited and advanced following each pedicle division as the uterine descent progressed. Bivalve and wedge morcellation proceeded slowly and methodically as the dominant myoma bulk was anterior located. Following uterine delivery, both adnexa were easily accessed for ovarian inspection and bilateral salpingectomy.

Recovery from the hysterectomy itself was routinely brisk. The unfortunate complication of peroneal neuropathy obviously was a huge setback to the overall recovery course, causing frustration and worry until fortunately symptoms completely dissipated. Low BMI, smoking, metal "candy cane" stirrups, and surgery greater than 4 hours are traditional factors all believed to increase likelihood for a compression neuropathy. This particular surgery involved none of those risks, as the patient was an overweight nonsmoker who was positioned in padded yellowfin stirrups and had an operative time under 4 hours.

LESSONS

- Nulliparity in combination with large myoma does not preclude VH
- Adnexa are usually accessible via vagina
- Complication can occur in any patient regardless of preoperative risk factors; a surgeon must be always vigilant.

CASE 9: MASSIVE DEBULKING OF KILOGRAM UTERUS WITH BILATERAL SALPINGECTOMY-1

Name: Mrs. SM
Age: 47 years
Parity: 2 FT normal vaginal delivery (FTND).
Indication for surgery: Mass effect, menorrhagia
Medical/surgical comorbidity: None
Operative time: 2 hours 30 min (inclusive of cystoscopy and uterosacral colposuspension).
Hemoglobin pre- and postoperative: 13 g/dL, 8.6 g/dL
Recovery course: Day 1 discharge, minimal pain, returns to work within 1 week.
Pathology report: Benign oviducts. Uterus 1,025 g, leiomyoma (add 10% to uterine weight, specimen sent directly in formalin to pathology. Gross weight directly in OR would be 10–15% more).
Preoperative evaluation: Patient with longstanding above symptoms and has reached point where they are no longer tolerable. Employed as nanny. Job entails frequent lifting. She has avoided surgery for years because she feared losing her job. Came to office on referral from friend in hope of a vaginal operation that will relieve her symptoms without long recuperation and missed work time.

Office evaluation involved pelvic examination revealing accessible cervix and mobile 18-week uterus. Benign endometrial biopsy was obtained. Office sonogram revealed favorable AP and transverse uterine dimensions at level of the lower uterine segment, suggestive of feasible vaginal access to uterine arteries. Patient counseled extensively and consented to "Trial VH" with possibility laparotomy.

What deters/dissuades: Large uterus.

Surgery: Routine sharp initial entry anteriorly to VUS and posterior to POD. Stepwise pedicle division followed after each step with return anteriorly to advance the vesicouterine dissection. In this case, despite large uterine size, following cardinal ligament division the anterior peritoneal reflection was identified and sharp anterior cul-de-sac entry was achieved. Uterine morcellation was methodical. Techniques of bivalve plus wedge resection plus myoma enucleation were all employed to gain descent and facilitate specimen delivery. Adnexa were both readily accessible for bilateral salpingectomy and ovarian inspection.

LESSONS

- Uterine size does not necessarily correlate with procedure difficulty. Shape of uterus, descent, mobility, presence of adenomyosis, fibroid number and fibroid consistency all factor into equation. One should not be dissuaded from attempting a large uterus when preoperative exam findings point to a favorable outcome
- Adnexa are accessible vaginally most of the time.

CASE 10: MASSIVE DEBULKING OF KILOGRAM UTERUS WITH BILATERAL SALPINGECTOMY-2

Name: Mrs. YC
Age: 50 years
Parity: 3 SVD
Indication for surgery: Mass effect, menorrhagia
Medical/surgical co morbidity: None
Operative time: 3 hours (inclusive of cystoscopy and uterosacral colposuspension).
Hemoglobin pre- and postoperative: 12.1 g/dL, 9 g/dL.
Recovery course: Day 1 discharge, uneventful rapid recovery.
Pathology report: Benign oviducts, uterus 1,097 g, adenomyosis, leiomyoma (add 10% to uterine weight, specimen sent directly in formalin to pathology. Gross weight directly in OR would be 10–15% more).
Preoperative evaluation: Benign endometrial biopsy. Cervix descends to hymen with traction. Roomy pelvis. Uterus mobile, but fills entire pelvis.
What deters/dissuades: Uterine size.
Surgery: Massive size of uterus anteriorly displaced bladder, complicating clear identification VUS dissection plane. Moderate bleeding encountered early on as initial anterior dissection was too deep, slightly below uterine serosa. After cardinal ligament division bleeding was addressed and proper dissection plane entered. Morcellation took slightly more than 1 hour, employing techniques of bivalve and wedge resection. Adnexa both readily accessed for ovarian inspection and salpingectomy.

LESSONS

- Large uterus should not dissuade Trial VH when exam is overall favorable
- Routine VH is known to be faster surgery with less blood loss than abdominal surgery. But very large, difficult VH can often take longer than abdominal surgery, and time required to morcellate uterine bulk can involve slow oozing blood loss that adds up. These concerns should not deter. Overall patient recovery is so much enhanced vaginally, and blood products are only rarely necessary even in long cases
- Accessibility of adnexa vaginally is the normal finding at VH.

CASE 11: DEBULKING OF LARGE ADENOMYOMA, BILATERAL SALPINGECTOMY-1

Name: Mrs. AK
Age: 44 years
Parity: Preterm SVD twins (largest 1,190 g).
Indication for surgery: Mass effect, menorrhagia.
Medical/surgical comorbidity: Smoker × 25 years.
Operative time: 3 hours (inclusive of cystoscopy and uterosacral colposuspension).
Hemoglobin pre- and postoperative: 12.7 g/dL, 11 g/dL.
Recovery course: Discharged home on day of surgery from recovery room, uneventful recovery, return to work in less than 2 weeks.
Pathology report: Benign oviducts. Uterus 515 g, adenomyosis and leiomyoma (add 10% to uterine weight, specimen sent directly in formalin to pathology. Gross weight directly in OR would be 10–15% more).
Preoperative evaluation: Patient a school teacher with longstanding above issues that are now intolerable. While she desperately wanted definitive management for her symptoms with surgery, she must be available to return to work at start of new school year – which begins in less than 2 weeks.

Mobile uterus, accessible cervix, benign endometrial biopsy all noted preoperatively. Patient appropriately counseled for "Trial VH", possible laparotomy.
What deters/dissuades: Uterine bulk, limited vaginal space and descent.

Surgery: Dominant anterior myoma and left adnexal adhesions combined to impede uterine descent for morcellation. This extended the total operative time in an otherwise uneventful operation. Due to the presence of adenomyosis the technique of morcellation employed was intramyometrial coring plus wedge resection. A large amount of dark blood noted intramyometrial during coring was consistent with the adenomyosis diagnosis. The right adnexa were easily accessed for ovarian inspection and salpingectomy. The left adnexa undescended due to adhesions. The oviduct was not visible or accessible. The left ovary was visible but relatively inaccessible with anterior and lateral adhesions.

LESSONS

- Adnexa in most cases are accessible. In reproductive age females, inaccessible adnexa are usually caused by pelvic adhesions
- Same day discharge is feasible following VH in select cases
- Surgeons interested in difficult VH cases should try to familiarize themselves with various vaginal morcellation techniques. Uterine pathology encountered at surgery can vary, and the surgeon armed with a varied approach to morcellation is in best position to adapt successfully.

CASE 12: DEBULKING OF LARGE ADENOMYOMA, BILATERAL SALPINGECTOMY-2

Name: Mrs. VI
Age: 45 years
Parity: 1 SVD
Indication for surgery: Mass effect, menorrhagia, dysmenorrhea, anemia.
Medical/surgical co morbidity: None
Operative time: 3 hours (inclusive of cystoscopy and uterosacral colposuspension).
Hemoglobin pre- and postoperative: 9.6 g/dL, 8.4 g/dL.
Recovery course: Day 1 discharge, uneventful rapid return to activity.
Pathology report: Benign oviducts. Uterus 463 g, adenomyosis, leiomyoma (add 10% to uterine weight, specimen sent directly in formalin to pathology. Gross weight directly in OR would be 10–15% more).
Preoperative evaluation: Patient with mass effect, pain and excessive bleeding. On exam the cervix was readily accessed vaginally and the large uterus was mobile with predominant anterior bulk. Endometrial biopsy was benign. Hemoglobin during the month prior to surgery increased from 6.7 to 9.6 with iron supplementation. Consent was for Trial VH due to concerns of starting low hemoglobin and an anticipated difficult morcellation.

Hemoglobin 6.7 g/dL 1 month prior to surgery. She increased to 9.6 g/dL with supplementation. Benign endometrial biopsy. Uterus mobile, large anterior fibroid amass, cervix readily accessed vaginally. Patient consented to Trial VH.
What deters/dissuades: Uterine size.
Surgery: Uncomplicated access to VUS anterior and VUS anteriorly and POD posteriorly, and division of lateral pedicles through uterine arteries. Size and shape of uterus complicated removal. Morcellation with bivalve and wedge took 75 minutes, after which both adnexa easily accessed for ovarian inspection and bilateral salpingectomy.

LESSON

- Adenomyosis generally makes for more difficult VH than fibroids, but should not discourage attempt when exam is favorable.

CASE 13: LARGE DEBULKING WITH BILATERAL SALPINGECTOMY FOR RECURRENT POSTMENOPAUSE BLEEDING

Name: Mrs. TL
Age: 69 years
Parity: 2 SVD
Indication for surgery: Recurrent postmenopause bleeding × 1 year.
Medical/surgical co morbidity: None
Operative time: 3 hours 30 min (inclusive of cystoscopy and uterosacral colposuspension).
Hemoglobin pre- and postoperative: 13 g/dL, 9.5 g/dL.
Recovery course: Day 1 discharge, uneventful recovery.
Pathology report: Benign oviducts, complex endometrial hyperplasia with atypia, 587 g uterus with leiomyoma (add 10% to uterine weight, specimen sent directly in formalin to pathology. Gross weight directly in OR would be 10–15% more).
Preoperative evaluation: Despite negative endometrial biopsy, postmenopause bleeding is persistent. Surgery agreed upon as Trial VH, possible laparotomy. Uterus is mobile, cervix readily accessible.
What deters/dissuades: Uterine size.

Surgery: A marked elongated cervix was encountered with minimal descent of lower uterine segment. The cervix was amputated, allowing for slight better access to an anterior myoma that was located behind pubis. After a small amount of posterior myometrium was removed, wedge resection was begun anteriorly. Progressive slow progress from this point using wedge and bivalve eventually achieved delivery of specimen. Both adnexa were accessible for salpingectomy and inspection of ovaries.

LESSONS

- Even postmenopause, adnexa tend to be accessible vaginally
- This was a very difficult surgery. Access to the cardinal and uterine artery pedicles was impeded from the combination of cervix elongation and an undescended uterus wedged behind the pubis as a result of its large and predominantly anterior fibroid bulk. Comfort with various morcellation techniques allows for surgeon flexibility and an enhanced ability to successfully manage a tough case such as this.

CASE 14: EARLY DEBULKING WITH THE AID OF VASOPRESSIN

Name: Mrs. DT
Age: 51 years
Parity: SVD × 1
Indication for surgery: Mass effect, anemia, menorrhagia.
Medical/surgical comorbidity: None
Operative time: 3 hours 15 min (inclusive of cystoscopy and uterosacral colposuspension).
Hemoglobin pre- and postoperative: 8.2 g/dL, 8.7 g/dL (2 units PRBC transfused intraoperative).
Recovery course: Day 1 discharge, uneventful course.
Pathology report: Benign oviducts, uterus 515 g, adenomyosis, leiomyoma (add 10% to uterine weight, specimen sent directly in formalin to pathology. Gross weight directly in OR would be 10–15% more).
Preoperative evaluation: Longstanding complaints as above noted. Readily accessible cervix. Mobile uterus. Benign endometrial biopsy obtained. Patient counseled for Trial VH.
What deters/dissuades: Uterine size.

Surgery: Patient did not wish to delay surgery to try to increase Hg. As she started with Hb 8 g/dL decision was made to start 2 units PRBC early on in the surgery as prophylactic measure given anticipated surgery blood loss.

After cardinal division the access to uterine arteries was limited, but descent of uterus provided access to posterior wall myomas. After vasopressin injection and fibroid enucleation performed the uterine debulking was sufficient to achieve needed descent for clamping artery pedicles and routine morcellation with bivalve and wedge to complete specimen delivery. Both adnexa readily accessed for salpingectomy and ovarian inspection.

LESSONS

- In select situations, where one is ready to convert abdominally if warranted, one can inject vasopressin and start morcellation process prior to securing uterine arteries in order to facilitate access to those pedicles
- Adnexa are accessible in nearly all VH cases.

Section 2A

VAGINAL HYSTERECTOMY WITH HISTORY OF CAESAREAN SECTION(S)

"If you want to grow roses, you also have to water the thorns!"

CASES

Dr Shirish S Sheth

Introduction
Case 15: VH with Left Ovarian Cystectomy
Case 16: VH Plus Stress Urinary Incontinence (SUI) Repair
Case 17: VH with Uterine Debulking
Case 18: VH with Right Ovarian Cystectomy Plus ?Endometrial Hyperplasia
Case 19: VH with Left Salpingo-oophorectomy for Ovarian Endometrial Cyst in a Morbidly Obese Patient
Case 20: VH with BSO for Right Ovarian Endometriotic Cyst
Case 21: VH with BSO for Abnormal Uterine Bleeding (AUB) with History of Caesarean Sections and Rupture Uterus
Case 22: VH Plus Vaginal Cuff with BSO for Postmenopausal Bleeder in a Morbidly Obese and Diabetic Patient
Case 23: VH with Altered Approach to Vesicouterine Peritoneum (VUP)

Dr Seth Finkelstein

Case 24: VH in Heavy Cigarette Smoker with H/O Two Classical Caesarean Sections via Midline Vertical Laparotomy
Case 25: VH with Uterine Debulking Plus Bilateral Salpingectomy of Tubal Remnants after Four Caesarean Sections and No Vaginal Births
Case 26: VH Plus Bilateral Salpingectomy after One Caesarean and No Vaginal Births
Case 27: VH with Uterine Debulking after Six Midline Vertical Laparotomies (Five Caesarean Sections and One Ectopic Pregnancy) in a Morbidly Obese Cigarette Smoker

CASE 15: VH WITH LEFT OVARIAN CYSTECTOMY

Name: Mrs. X
Age: 47 years
Parity: 2 FTCS
H/O: No relevant history
Complains of (C/O): Heavy menses for 3 months followed by continuous bleeding since 45 days.

Clinically diagnosed as abnormal uterine bleeding (AUB) due to uterine adenomyosis. Endometrial hyperplasia and more to be ruled out.

Not obese. No history of (H/O) hypertension or diabetes. Uterus 12 weeks size, mobile with clear fornices. Favorable cervical descent to attempt VH.

Sonography confirmed normal abdominopelvic findings except for uterine volume of 300 cm^3 with 16 mm endometrial thickness.
Diagnosis: Uterine adenomyosis with ?E. hyperplasia.
Operation: VH with left ovarian cystectomy.
What deters/dissuades: Bladder separation.

Vaginal hysterectomy started as usual. Uterocervical-broad ligament space was used to access the VUP.[1-8]

Bladder was easily separated laterally and later medially. After uterines were secured, the cervix was well bisected to reach the lower uterine wall. Gentle, debulking was done by morcellation of the adenomyotic uterine walls and hysterectomy completed. Ovaries were normal and preserved except a small simple cyst in the left ovary was excised and healthy part 95% of the ovary was preserved. Uterus was sent for frozen histopathological (HP) study, which was negative for malignancy. The frozen section analysis should be done by experienced pathologists and the possible predictive factors affecting a false diagnosis should carefully be taken into consideration.[9] After checking hemostasis, vaginal closure was done. Blood transfusion was not needed. Hospital stay was 2 days with an uneventful speedy recovery (Figs. 1 to 6).

Histopathology reported uterus 320 g. Deep adenomyosis with left ovarian simple cyst. No malignancy.
What inspired: Lies in uterocervical-broad ligament space and frozen HP facility.

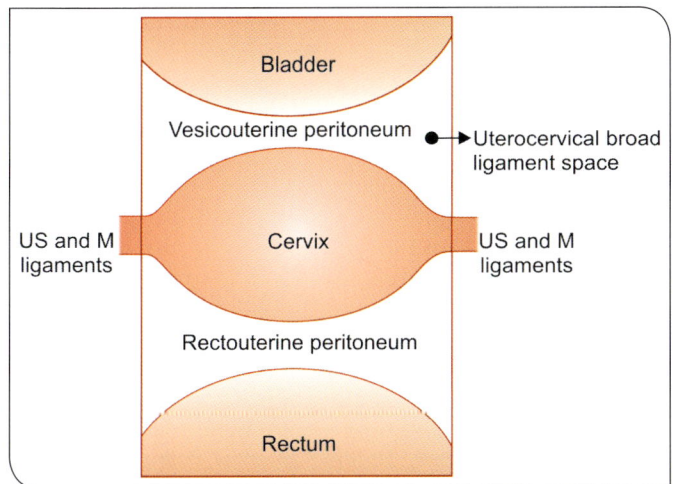

Fig. 1: This figure distinctly shows the space between bladder and cervix or cervicouterine surface, which is much more under lateral one-fifth of bladder when compared with central three-fifths of bladder.[4]

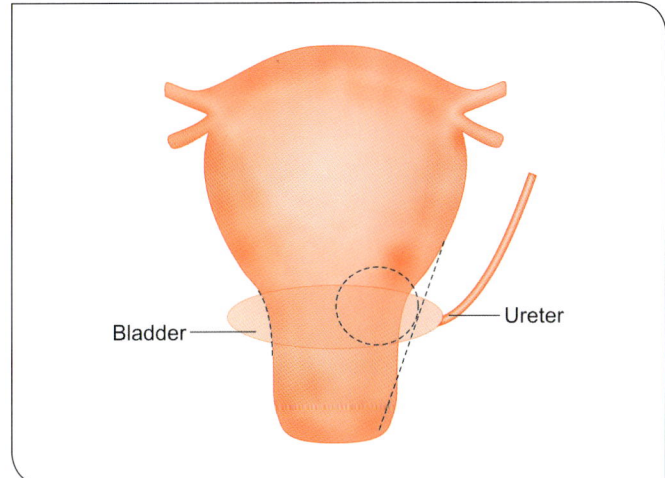

Fig. 2: Broad circle marks the site of the uterocervical-broad ligament space.[1,3]

INTRODUCTION

A mere history of (H/O) caesarean sections in the past is enough to inhibit many gynecologists from performing hysterectomy via the vaginal route.[1,2] These women are not even carefully examined in an unbiased manner and evaluated before they are taken for laparoscopic or abdominal hysterectomy. As such the incidence of abdominal hysterectomy is pathologically high, as if there is no concern about the well-being of women and this reflects a surgical weakness.

However, to have a history of rupture uterus per se is highly disturbing and inhibiting to even consider removal of such a uterus via the vaginal route. A rupture in the past added to a history of previous caesarean sections is even more daunting to consider vaginal hysterectomy (VH) because of the possibility of adhesions, difficulty in getting a plane of cleavage and a high risk of damaging the bladder and/or rectum and more.[3-7] However actually what counts is what are the clinical findings and do they contraindicate vaginal route for hysterectomy?

If cervix has physiological descent with a freely mobile uterus and clear fornices without adnexal pathology, there is no indication to open the abdomen or use a laparoscope. Rupture uterus being rare,[1] one may have apprehensions about the adhesions causing difficulty and complications. Thus, it is worth performing an evaluatory or diagnostic laparoscopy to confirm that pelvic findings will permit hysterectomy via the vaginal route. Besides examination under anesthesia, laparoscopy gives clear picture of the bladder, vesicouterine peritoneum (VUP), pouch of Douglas (POD) and the surroundings. Diagnostic laparoscopy adds abdominal invasion by only a single 5 mm puncture. Flimsy adhesions are meaningless to worry about. If the peritoneum is accessible from anterior and posterior, the rest is usually not difficult or to worry about even, if the uterus had ruptured in the past and created an emergency then.

Successful VH on such a rare case definitely instills extra confidence to operate on a similar rare case in the future. The ideal is to ask oneself that with given clinical findings in absence of a H/O caesarean section and rupture uterus in the past, would one have attempted VH or not? The answer should guide one's decision making.

Vaginal surgery particularly for getting an access to the VUP needs familiarity and friendliness with cervicovesical strands, urinary bladder, bladder pillars and surrounding tissues. Anatomically available lateral-free space, the uterocervical-broad ligament space, facilitates separation of the centrally adherent bladder.[3-8]

Once accessed, opening or cutting open of VUP is not vital even after reaching up to the uterine fundus. It is vital to have the bladder retractor between the uterocervical surface covered by a thin peritoneum posteriorly and the bladder anteriorly. Peritoneum may be cut or opened later. When possible, it is safer to intrude/invade from the accessible lateral, cornual end of the uterus by passing finger(s) from POD to the right or left nearer the cornual end and try to have the finger pushing the thin peritoneum to the front for one to appreciate and cut. This secures the space to expand so as to place the bladder retractor and keep the bladder upwards and away.

Once VH is possible, in a woman with past H/O caesarean section(s), debulking, prophylactic salpingo-oophorectomy or for adnexal pathology and endometrial cancer can be dealt with vaginally on its merits and operator's zeal and experience.

REFERENCES

1. Sheth SS. Results of treatment of rupture of the uterus by suturing. J Obstet Gynaec Brit Cwlth. 1968;75:55-8.
2. Sheth SS. Vaginal hysterectomy following earlier ruptured uterus and caesarean sections. J Gynecol Surg. 1998;14:185-9.
3. Sheth SS. Vaginal hysterectomy. In: Studd JW (Ed). Progress in Obstetrics and Gynecology, Volume 10, 1st edition. London, UK: Churchill Livingstone; 1992. pp. 317-40.
4. Sheth SS, Malpani AN. Vaginal hysterectomy following previous caesarean section. Int J Gynaecol Obstet. 1995;50(2):165-9.
5. Sheth SS. An approach to vesicouterine peritoneum through a new surgical space. J Gynecol Surg. 1996;12:135-40.
6. Sheth SS. Access to vesicouterine and rectouterine pouches. In: Sheth SS (Ed). Vaginal Hysterectomy, 2nd edition. New Delhi, India: Jaypee Brothers Medical Publishers (P) Ltd; 2014. pp. 31-50.
7. Sizzi O, Paparella P, Bonito C, et al. Laparoscopic assistance after vaginal hysterectomy and unsuccessful access to the ovaries or failed uterine mobilization: changing trends. JSLS. 2004;8(4):339-46.
8. Sheth SS. Observations from a FIGO Past President on vaginal hysterectomy and related surgery by the vaginal route. Int J Gynecol Obstet. 2016;135:1-4.

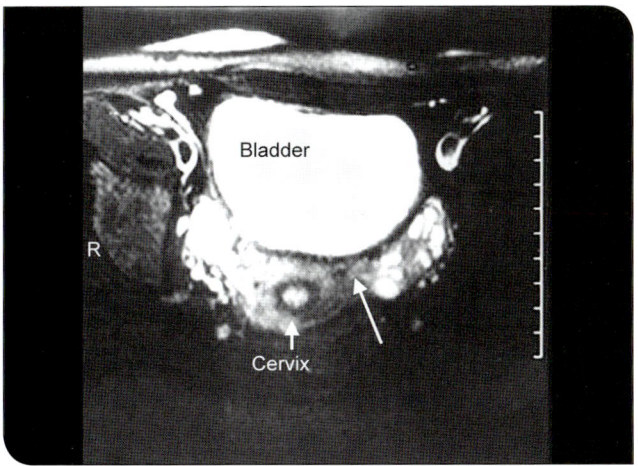

Fig. 3: Magnetic resonance imaging (MRI) study showing distinctly the presence of free space.[4]

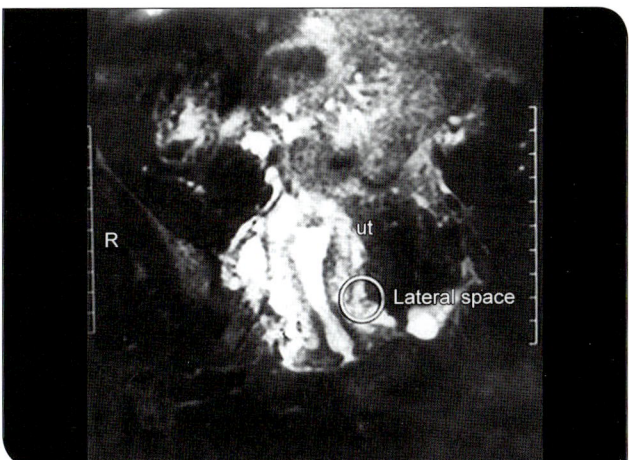

Fig. 4: MRI study confirming the presence of free-space surgical window (uterocervical-broad ligament space).[4]

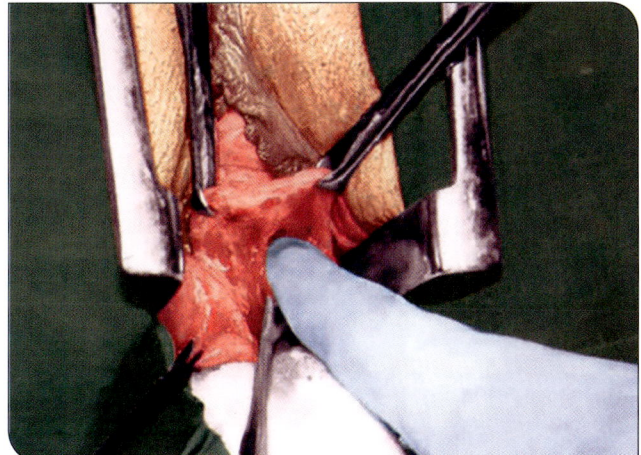

Fig. 5: The uterocervical-broad ligament space. The tip of the finger remains on the uterocervical surface, with the bladder anteromedially, as it insinuates further between the two leaves of the broad ligament.[4]

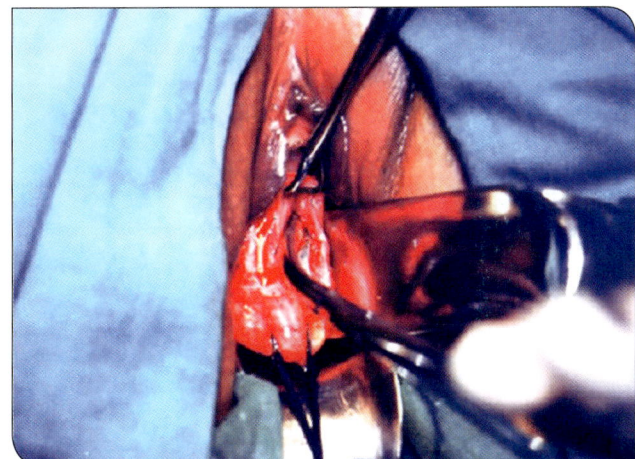

Fig. 6: The bladder is held with a Babcock's forceps, with an artery forceps in the uterocervical-broad ligament space.[4]

LESSONS

- In absence of history of caesarean sections in the past, with same clinical findings, would I have done VH? If answer is favorable, an attempt should be made to perform VH.

- Frozen HP study spared the patient from hysteroscopy plus dilatation and curettage (D&C) as well and more invasive abdominal access for hysterectomy.[10]

CASE 16: VH PLUS STRESS URINARY INCONTINENCE (SUI) REPAIR

Name: Mrs. X
Age: 50 years
Parity: 2 FTCS

Not obese. No H/O hypertension or diabetes; AUB, uterus 6 weeks size, volume 115 cm³; moderate stress urinary incontinence (SUI).

Diagnosis: AUB plus SUI.

Operation: VH followed by transvaginal obturator tape (TVTO).

Vaginal hysterectomy was performed as per routine, except for accessing the VUP the uterocervical-broad ligament space was utilized.[1-3] Naked eye examination revealed no endometrial pathology. Ovaries were preserved. TVTO was done for SUI.[11-13] Hemostasis was checked and vaginal closure done. Blood transfusion was not needed. Hospital stay was 2 days followed by an uneventful speedy recovery. Abdomen remained intact (Fig. 1).

Histopathology showed uterus weight 120 g. Deep adenomyosis with fibroid. Atypical squamous metaplasia with basal hyperplasia. No malignancy.

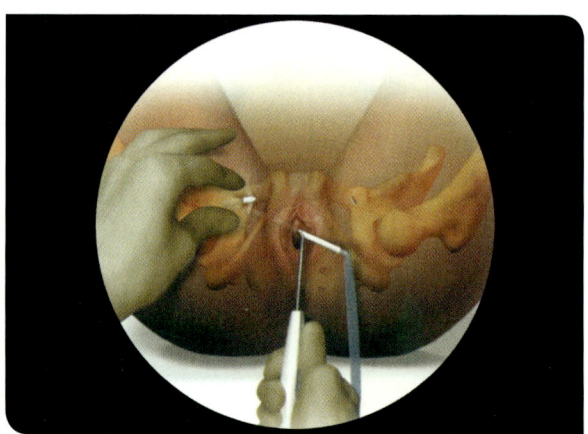

Fig. 1: Transvaginal obturator tape (TVTO) for tension-free support (Gynecare TVT obturator system).

LESSON

- Spares from an additional visit to the operation theater (room) by combining TVTO with VH in a patient with or without a H/O two caesarean sections in the past. TVTO added flavor to VH after two caesarean sections in past.

CASE 17: VH WITH UTERINE DEBULKING

Name: Mrs. X
Age: 46 years
Parity: 3 FTCS
Last delivery (LD): 22 years back
C/O: Heavy menses since 2 months.

Not obese. No H/O hypertension or diabetes.

Uterus was 14 weeks size, nodular with favorable cervical descent to attempt VH. Fornices were clear.

Sonography revealed 11 cm × 8.9 cm × 6.3 cm with fundal fibroid of 5.1 cm. Uterus volume 333 cm³. Adnexae normal.

Diagnosis: Uterine fibroids.
Operation: VH with debulking.
What deters/dissuades: H/O three caesarean sections in the past.

Vaginal hysterectomy started as usual. VUP was accessed with the help of uterocervical-broad ligament space[1,2,4] (Fig. 1). Uterines were secured and the cervix bisected as high as possible and uterus was debulked by morcellation and enucleation to complete VH.[14-17] She did not require more dissection despite H/O three caesarean sections in the past.[18,19] Healthy tubes and ovaries were preserved. Hemostasis was checked and vaginal closure done.

Blood transfusion was not needed. Hospital stay was 2 days. Postoperatively, she had an uneventful speedy recovery.

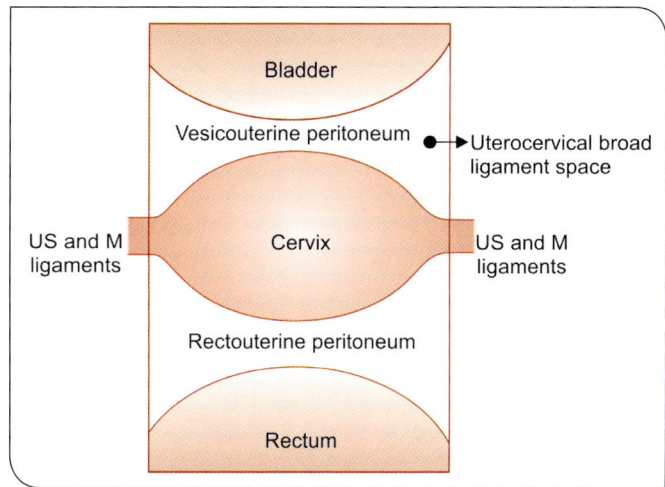

Fig. 1: Distinctly shows the space between bladder and cervix or cervicouterine surface, which is much more under lateral one-fifth of bladder when compared with central three-fifths of bladder.[4]

Histopathology: Uterus 14 weeks size, weighed 420 g. Leiomyomatous with severe adenomyosis. No malignancy.
What inspired: Utereocervical broad ligament space plus experience of debulking paved the way.

LESSON

- The patient was spared a fourth opening of the abdomen OR 5 abdominal cuts.

CASE 18: VH WITH RIGHT OVARIAN CYSTECTOMY PLUS ?ENDOMETRIAL HYPERPLASIA

Name: Mrs. X
Age: 49 years
Parity: 1st FTCS, 2nd FTND
Last delivery (LD): 18 years back
C/O: Spotting per vaginam followed by heavy bleeding since 2 months.
 Not obese. No H/O hypertension or diabetes.
Diagnosis: Uterine fibroids with ?Endometrial hyperplasia plus right ovarian cyst.
Operation: VH with right ovarian cystectomy.
 Clinically uterus 14 weeks size, cervix with physiological descent with clear fornices.
 Sonography showed 13 cm × 9 cm × 7 cm, volume 442 cm³, endometrial thickness 20 mm. Right ovary—follicular cyst of 2 cm.
 Bladder was separated with the help of uterocervical-broad ligament space[1-3] (Fig. 1). Morcellation plus enucleation helped to complete the VH.[16,17,19] Uterus was sent for frozen HP study. Reported complex hyperplasia, no CANCER or ATYPIA.[15,20] Right ovarian cystectomy of 2 cm × 2 cm was done.[21,22] Healthy ovaries were preserved. For right fimbrial cyst and paratubal cyst, right salpingectomy was done and hysterectomy completed.
 Hemostasis was checked and vaginal closure done. Blood transfusion was not needed. Hospital stay was 2 days followed by an uneventful speedy recovery.
Histopathology: Uterus weighed 435 g. Leiomyomata, severe adenomyosis. Right tube normal. Ovarian and paratubal cysts nothing abnormal. Right ovarian simple cyst. No malignancy.
What inspired: Uterocervical-broad ligament space and experience of adnexal pathology at VH.

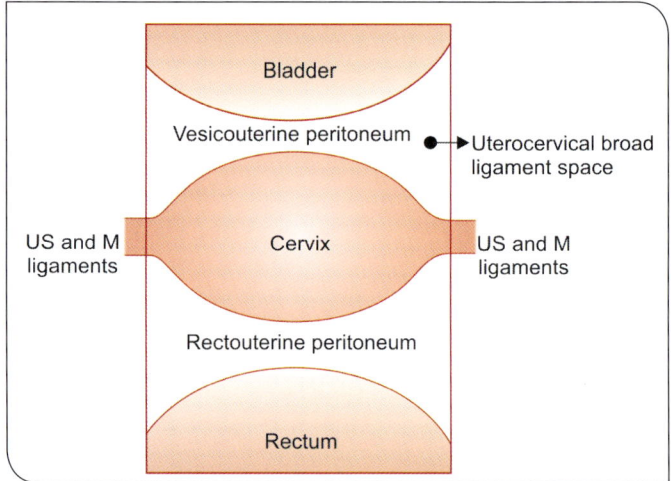

Fig. 1: Distinctly shows the space between bladder and cervix or cervicouterine surface, which is much more under lateral one-fifth of bladder when compared with central three-fifths of bladder.[4]

LESSONS

- Frozen HP study spared the patient from hysteroscopy plus D&C and more invasive abdominal access.
- Debulking added flavor.

CASE 19: VH WITH LEFT SALPINGO-OOPHORECTOMY FOR OVARIAN ENDOMETRIAL CYST IN A MORBIDLY OBESE PATIENT

Name: Mrs. X
Age: 38 years
Parity: 2 FTCS
C/O: Heavy and painful menses.

Morbidly obese [body mass index (BMI) 42]. No H/O hypertension or diabetes.

Uterus 10+ weeks size, cervix with physiological descent to attempt VH and left ovarian cyst endometriotic. Right and posterior fornices were clear. Sonography confirmed an enlarged uterus with 180 cm^3 volume and left ovarian endometrial cyst of 6.6 cm × 5.8 cm × 4.3 cm.

Diagnosis: Uterine adenomyosis plus left ovarian endometrial cyst in a morbidly obese patient[23-26] (Figs. 1 to 3).
Operation: VH with left salpingo-oophorectomy plus right salpingectomy. Taken as "trial vaginal route" case.[2,14]
What deters/dissuades: Likely adhesions.

For VH, access to the VUP was via the uterocervical-broad ligament space.[1-4] POD was accessed with extra care[4] and difficulty and hysterectomy was completed. Cut open uterus showed normal endometrium. Left ovary was low down and when held firmly with Babcock forceps, poured chocolaty material for which left salpingo-oophorectomy was performed.[21,22] Prophylactic right salpingectomy was done.[27] Right healthy ovary was preserved as she was very keen to have it preserved (Age: 38 years). Hemostasis was checked and vaginal closure done. Blood transfusion was not needed. Hospital stay was 2 days followed by an uneventful speedy recovery.

Histopathology showed uterus weighed 213 g with severe adenomyosis. Left ovarian endometriotic cyst and both tubes are normal. No evidence of malignancy.

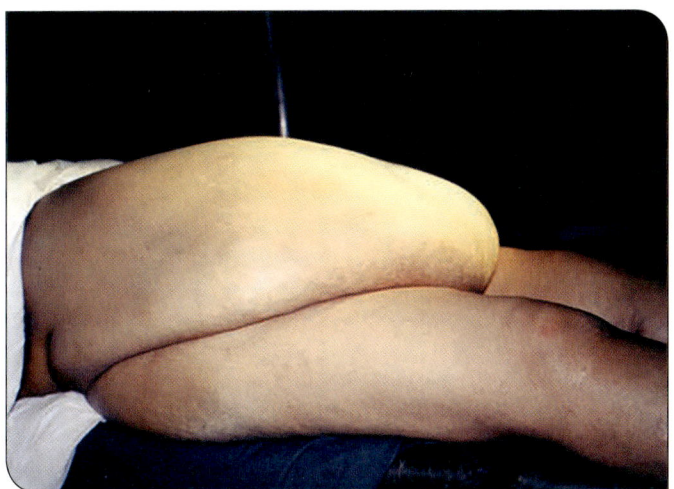

Fig. 1: Obese woman. Obesity favors vaginal route.[23]

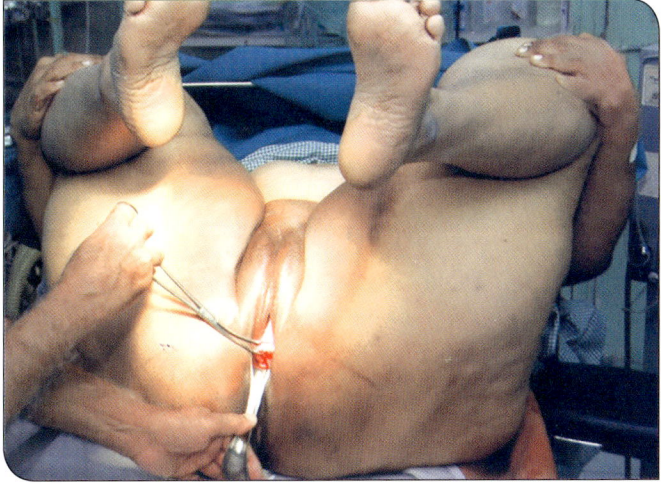

Fig. 2: Superflexion position. The patient's hands keep both feet apart and thus provide a clear view of the vulva and vaginal area.
Source: Adapted from Seth SS. Superflexion position for difficult speculum examination. Int J Gynaecol Obstet. 2013;121:92-3.

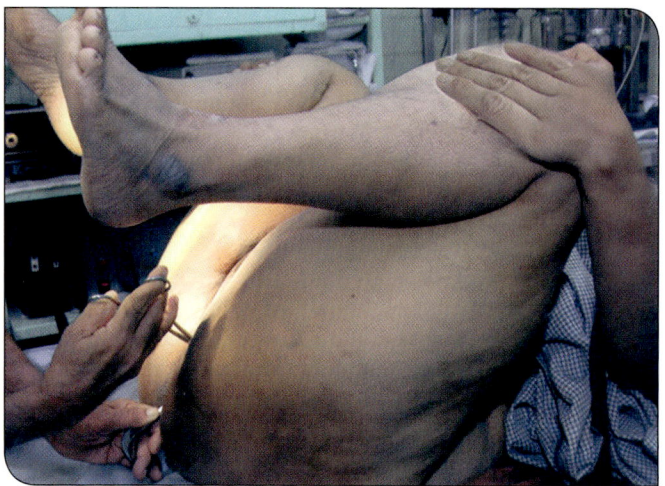

Fig. 3: The patient's both hands are keeping her both feet apart and thus providing clear view of the vulva vaginal area and required speculum examination.[15]

What inspired: Uterocervical-broad ligament space and experience of salpingo-oophorectomy for adnexal pathology at VH in obese women.

LESSONS

- Vaginal route is possible in a morbidly obese patient with H/O caesarean sections in the past.
- Sizeable endometriotic cyst added flavor.

CASE 20: VH WITH BSO FOR RIGHT OVARIAN ENDOMETRIOTIC CYST

Name: Mrs. X
Age: 50 years
Parity: 2 FTCS
LD: 18 years back.
C/O: Prolonged, heavy and painful menses.
H/O: Laparoscopic surgery for right ovarian endometriosis.
　Normal size uterus with restricted mobility. Cervix: Healthy with physiological descent to attempt vaginal hysterectomy. Lateral and posterior fornices had tender firm mass. 'Dimple Sign' absent.[21,28-30] This was later confirmed under anesthesia.
Sonography: Uterus volume 100 cm³, right ovary with 3 cm × 2 cm endometriotic cyst. Right tube and left ovary were normal. Left tubal hydrosalpinx.
Diagnosis: Right ovarian endometrial cyst with left tubal hydrosalpinx.
Operation: VH with bilateral salpingo-oophorectomy (BSO).
What deters/dissuades: Endometriotic ovarian cyst.
Anterior peritoneum was accessed with the help of uterocervical broad ligament space[1-4] (Fig. 1). Access to posterior peritoneum via pouch of Douglas was carefully separated keeping soft tissue away from the posterior cervico-uterine surface and feel firm posterior cervicouterine surface directly and get an access to the peritoneum from the posterior space.[4,21,31] Access was confirmed by pouring of chocolaty material. Escape of chocolaty material or fluid from POD is a good sign – a highly satisfying one (Figs. 2 to 5).

Uterus was totally bisected from the cervix till the fundus to deal with each adnexectomy with the help of traction on hemihysterectomized or half uterus.[21,22] Right tube and right ovary were adherent to the surrounding tissues. Left ovary was normal. After adhesiolysis, tube and ovary were freed on right for salpingo-oophorectomy. Traction on the hemihysterectomized uterus felicitated access to right infundibulopelvic ligament after cutting the round ligament as laterally as possible. Thenafter, left salpingo-oophorectomy was easily done, including left hydrosalpinx. No endometriotic tissue was seen in the operative field. Hysterectomy with BSO was completed. Cut open uterus showed normal endometrium. Hemostasis was checked and closure done. Blood transfusion was not needed. Hospital stay was 2 days followed by an uneventful speedy recovery.

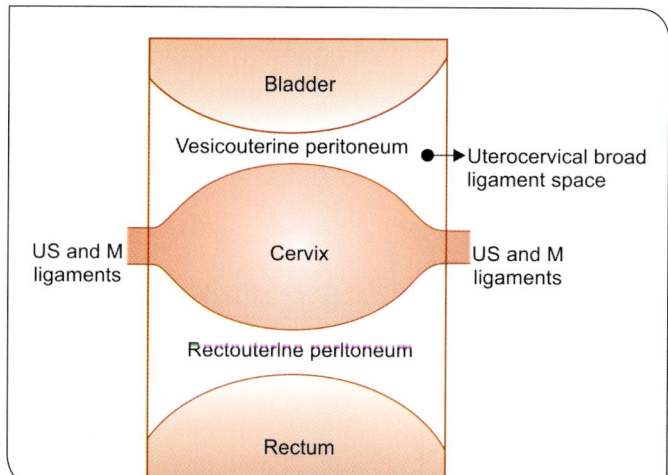

Fig. 1: Distinctly shows the space between bladder and cervix or cervicouterine surface, which is much more under lateral one-fifth of bladder when compared with central three-fifths of bladder.[4]

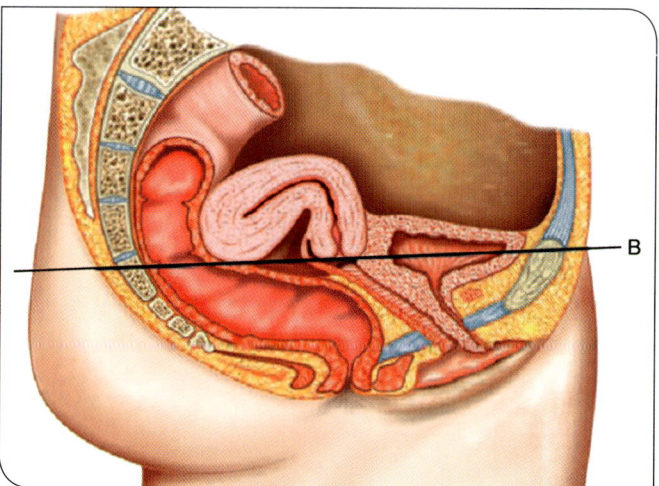

Fig. 2: A marked retroversion with retroflexion creates a space between the uterocervical junction and the B line.
Source: Prepared by surgeon, Dr RD Prabhu, Shimoga, Karnataka, India.[31]

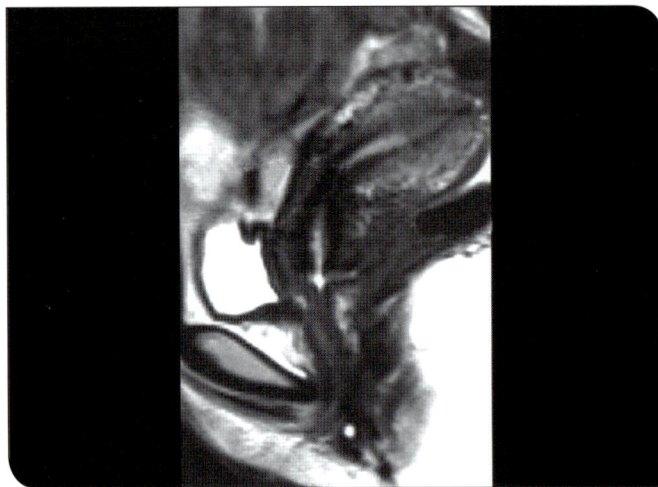

Fig. 3: MRI showing a retroverted and retroflexed uterus as well as the posterior uterocervical-broad ligament space, which measured 1.36 cm vertically and 0.73 cm transversally.
Source: MRI prepared by Dr Nilesh Shah and Dr Manjari Bapat, Mumbai, Maharashtra, India.[31]

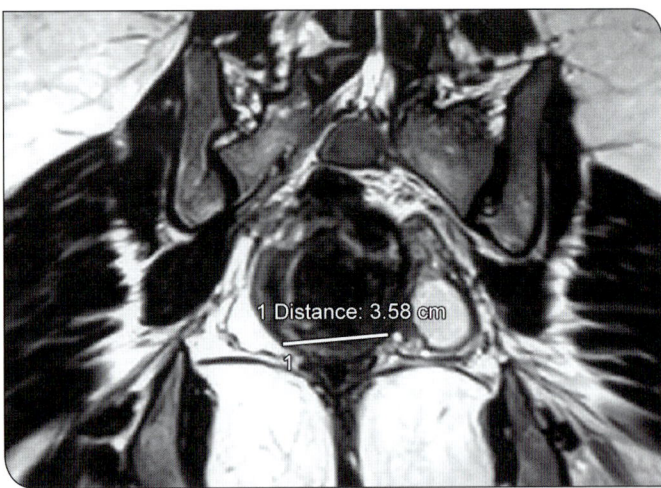

Fig. 4: MRI showing the width of the transverse posterior uterocervical-broad ligament space; it is the width of the uterocervical junction, plus 1 cm to the broad ligament on both sides.
Source: MRI prepared by Dr Nilesh Shah and Dr Manjari Bapat, Mumbai, Maharashtra, India.[31]

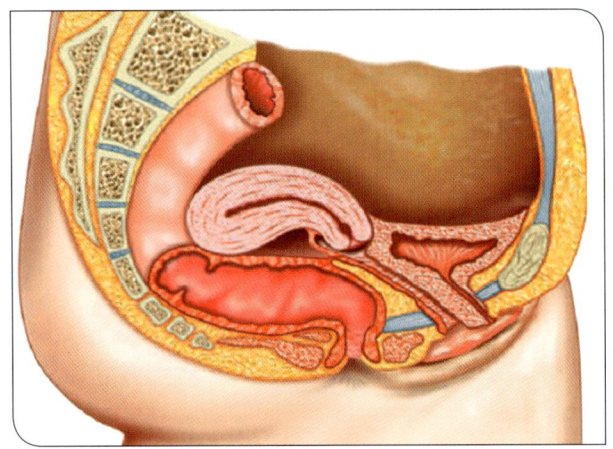

Fig. 5: Adherent mass in the posterior uterocervical-broad ligament space.
Source: Prepared by surgeon, Dr RD Prabhu, Shimoga, Karnataka, India.[31]

Histopathology revealed normal uterus, severe right ovarian endometriosis and normal right tube and left ovary. Left tube with hydrosalpinx. No malignancy.

What inspired?
1. Experience of dealing with obliterated POD and ovarian endometriosis.
2. Endometrial cyst was not large.
3. Taken as 'Trial vaginal route' case.

LESSON

- Contraindication did not deter.

What adds flavor: H/O Caesarean Section in the past.

CASE 21: VH WITH BSO FOR ABNORMAL UTERINE BLEEDING (AUB) WITH HISTORY OF CAESAREAN SECTIONS AND RUPTURE UTERUS

Name: Mrs. X
Age: 41 years
Parity: 4 (1st, 3rd and 4th FTCS and 2nd rupture uterus).

She had her first confinement by caesarean section followed by a ruptured uterus in the lower uterine segment during her second pregnancy for which the uterus was sutured and preserved.[32,33] Following the rupture of the uterus in the past, she had two elective caesarean sections for her next two pregnancies (Fig. 1). At the time of the last one she underwent tubal sterilization.

She now had 8 weeks size uterus with menorrhagia not responding to medical treatment and H/O three D&Cs which had showed a benign endometrium. In between, the hemoglobin had fallen to 6.5 g. She was keen to have her uterus removed and not have abdominal surgery again.

Earlier it was explained to her that she could have a long-acting intrauterine device (IUD) or endometrial ablation to avoid surgery. She was even offered laparoscopic bilateral oophorectomy but she declined that, as well as opening of the abdomen for hysterectomy. She requested and pleaded for hysterectomy via the vaginal route to spare her abdominal surgery. In fact, she said that she travelled to Bombay (Mumbai) from a small place in Gujarat state to avoid abdominal surgery. This was the inspiration to attempt a hysterectomy via the vaginal route in such a rare case and to establish the credibility of the route and technique.

Clinically, there was a freely mobile 8 weeks size uterus without pelvic pathology, i.e. labeled as dysfunctional uterine bleeding in the past. Sonography showed a uterus volume of 130 cm³, adenomyotic with other normal findings. The same was confirmed under anesthesia and a decision taken to do hysterectomy by the vaginal route.

I asked myself, in absence of the previously ruptured uterus and H/O caesarean sections in the past and based on the findings at clinical examination and examination under anesthesia, would I have attempted VH? If the answer was yes, one can attempt a hysterectomy via the vaginal route as a "trial VH" case.[2,14]

However this being rare and unreported earlier in the literature, in case any complication occurred because of the VH, the blame and universal comment would be "Why was laparoscopic or abdominal hysterectomy not done?"

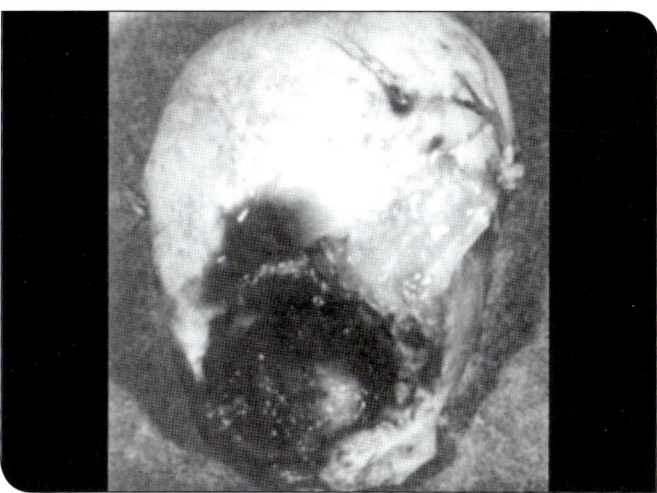

Fig. 1: Rupture of uterus identified immediately after vaginal delivery; the previous delivery was by caesarean section with a vertical uterine incision.
Source: Adapted from "In: Pritchard JA, MacDonald PC, Gant NF (Eds). William's Obstetrics, 17th edition. USA: A Publishing Division of Prentice Hall Incorporation; 1985. pp. 697-706".

Therefore, evaluatory or diagnostic laparoscopy was performed to get a crystal clear picture of the interior to avoid complications. Laparoscopic evaluation found nothing contraindicating the vaginal route and boosted my confidence to undertake VH.

Diagnosis: AUB (?adenomyosis) with past history of rupture uterus and caesarean sections.
Operation: VH with BSO.
What deters/dissuades: H/O rupture of the uterus in the past.

Vaginal hysterectomy was performed without difficulty. Because of three caesarean sections and a ruptured uterus on one occasion, the VUP or the bladder separation was achieved via the uterocervical-broad ligament space[1-4] and hysterectomy completed as per routine[34] (Fig. 2). Advantageously, access to VUP was easy. The patient was very keen to have her ovaries removed and have no more surgeries in life, particularly of the genital tract. Therefore, concomitant BSO was performed at her request. Hemostasis was checked and vaginal closure done.

Blood loss was less than 50 mL. She had an uneventful speedy recovery from the surgery and went home after 24 hours. Postoperative follow-up showed excellent results.

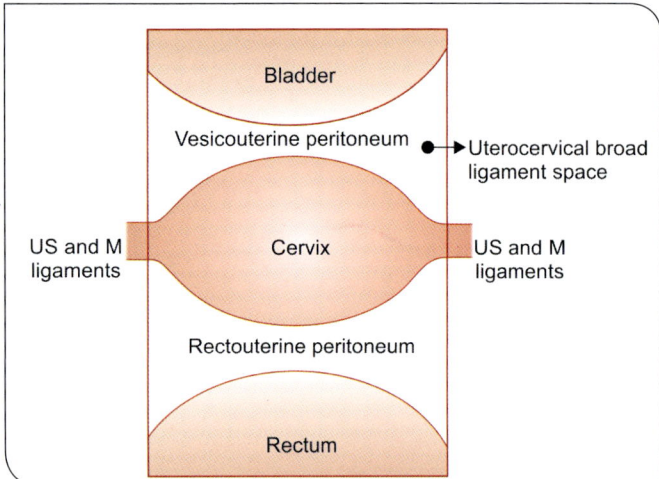

Fig. 2: Distinctly shows the space between bladder and cervix or cervicouterine surface, which is much more under lateral one-fifth of bladder when compared with central three-fifths of bladder.[4]

Histopathology showed a uterus that weighed 160 g with severe adenomyosis, with normal tubes and ovaries. No malignancy.

It is worth keeping in mind that 80% of the world does not have a laparoscope and/or laparoscopist and a woman may refuse any more opening of the abdomen.[30] Fortunately, rupture of the uterus is so rare in the affluent world and consideration of vaginal route for hysterectomy for such past history is more rare.

Kovac et al.[35] suggest laparoscopically-assisted vaginal hysterectomy (LAVH) for gaining entry through a scarred anterior *cul-de-sac* after caesarean section. Coulam and Pratt[36] believe that the chief concern centers on bladder injury and difficulty in gaining entry through the scarred anterior *cul-de-sac*. Hoffman and Jaeger[37] mention that a history of multiple caesarean sections has been considered a relative contraindication to hysterectomy via the vaginal route. Inadvertent injury to the bladder is likely to increase with the rising number of caesarean sections in the past. The adhesions between the bladder and the lower uterine segment, particularly after caesarean section in the past can be dense or tough in the midline but not laterally.[1,4] Let a H/O caesarean section not be taken as an excuse to avoid VH. Entry from the free-lateral space, i.e. uterocervical-broad ligament space can pave the way.[38] However, adhesions following ruptured uterus is unknown or anyone's guess. Therefore a diagnostic laparoscopy was performed.

What inspired
- The patient's desperate plea to keep the abdomen intact inspired to undertake VH.
- With same clinical findings in the absence of past H/O caesarean sections and rupture uterus, I would have done VH.
- Zeal to meet the challenge of rarity to undertake VH.

LESSON
- Rare opportunity explored.

CASE 22: VH PLUS VAGINAL CUFF WITH BSO FOR POSTMENOPAUSAL BLEEDER IN A MORBIDLY OBESE AND DIABETIC PATIENT

Name: Mrs. X
Age: 53 years
Parity: 1 FTCS
C/O: Heavy menses for 3 months followed by continuous bleeding for 40 days.

Clinically diagnosed as AUB due to ?endometrial hyperplasia. Morbidly obese (BMI: 44), hypertensive and diabetic with 10 weeks size uterus, healthy cervix and clear fornices. Favorable physiological descent of cervix to attempt VH (Fig. 1).

Sonography showed normal abdominal pelvic findings except uterine volume of 130 cm^3 with 24 mm endometrial thickness.

Diagnosis: ?Endometrial hyperplasia, endometrial malignancy.

Operation: VH with vaginal cuff plus BSO.

Vaginal hysterectomy started with a vaginal cuff of 3 cm. Access to VUP was through uterocervical-broad ligament space because of caesarean section in the past.[1,2] Because of obesity, she needed extra traction on the cervix as well as extra retraction of the lateral vaginal walls.[23,24,26] Soon after hysterectomy, intraoperatively, the uterus was sent for frozen HP study. Meanwhile, BSO was completed.[21] Frozen HP reported well-differentiated adenocarcinoma with 0.7 cm invasion of myometrial wall out of 2.3 cm. This was freely discussed with the patient's husband as she did not require lymph node removal and hence no further surgery.[14,19,20] Preoperatively, the patient had been fully informed and counseled about frozen HP study and requiring necessary treatment with informed consent. She preferred frozen HP study to avoid an extra visit to operation theater/room (OT/OR) for hysteroscopy plus D&C and was keen to have the ovaries removed.

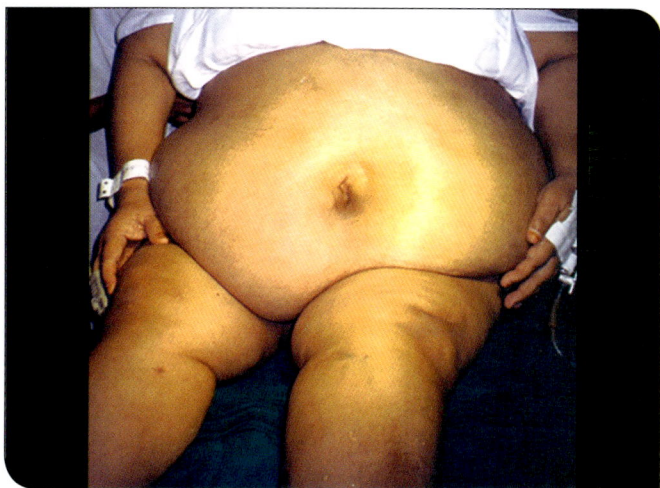

Fig. 1: Obese woman. Obesity favors vaginal route.[14]

After checking hemostasis, vaginal closure was done. Blood transfusion was not needed. Hospital stay was 2 days with a speedy uneventful recovery.

Histopathology reported uterus of 160 g, well-differentiated endometrioid adenocarcinoma with 7 mm myometrial invasion of wall out of 23 mm.

What inspired: Facility for frozen HP study and readiness to switch over to abdominal route.

LESSON

- VH in a morbidly obese, hypertensive and diabetic patient with H/O caesarean section. This spared her from hysteroscopy plus curettage earlier and also abdominal approach for hysterectomy with greater invasion as well as morbidity.

CASE 23: VH WITH ALTERED APPROACH TO VESICOUTERINE PERITONEUM (VUP)

Name: Mrs. X
Age: 43 years
Parity: 3 FTCS
H/O: No relevant history.
C/O: Heavy menses for 6 months.

Not obese. No H/O hypertension or diabetes.

Uterus 10 weeks size, healthy cervix with physiological descent and clear fornices. Sonography confirmed normal pelvic findings except uterine volume being 180 cm^3 with endometrial thickness of 18 mm. Recent H/O hysteroscopy plus curettage showed complex hyperplasia without atypia.

Diagnosis: ?Adenomyosis with endometrial hyperplasia.
Operation: VH with prophylactic bilateral salpingectomy.
What deters/dissuades: H/O three caesarean sections in the past.

Vaginal hysterectomy started as usual. Uterocervical-broad ligament space was used to separate the bladder from laterally. However, the bladder was densely-adherent centrally and it needed extra care to reach the higher uterine serosa laterally. After uterines were secured, reached little higher but that was not adequate for full separation of the bladder. Since bladder separation was risky, the cervix was bisected to debulk the uterus and draw fundus and cornual area closer for an access to separate the bladder. Traction was applied on the posterior uterine wall to bring out the uterus partially from free space posteriorly. It was then possible for a finger to reach right cornual area via POD or from posterior-free space. This facilitated the finger to appear anteriorly but covered with thin peritoneum. Thin peritoneum was cut for a finger to enter and thus make space. The space was widened to put the bladder retractor.[18] This also permitted severance of the right upper pedicle and free the uterus totally on the right side. This was adequate to complete the hysterectomy vaginally. Ovaries were found normal. They were preserved and only bilateral partial salpingectomy done (Flow chart 1). After checking hemostasis, vaginal closure was done. Blood

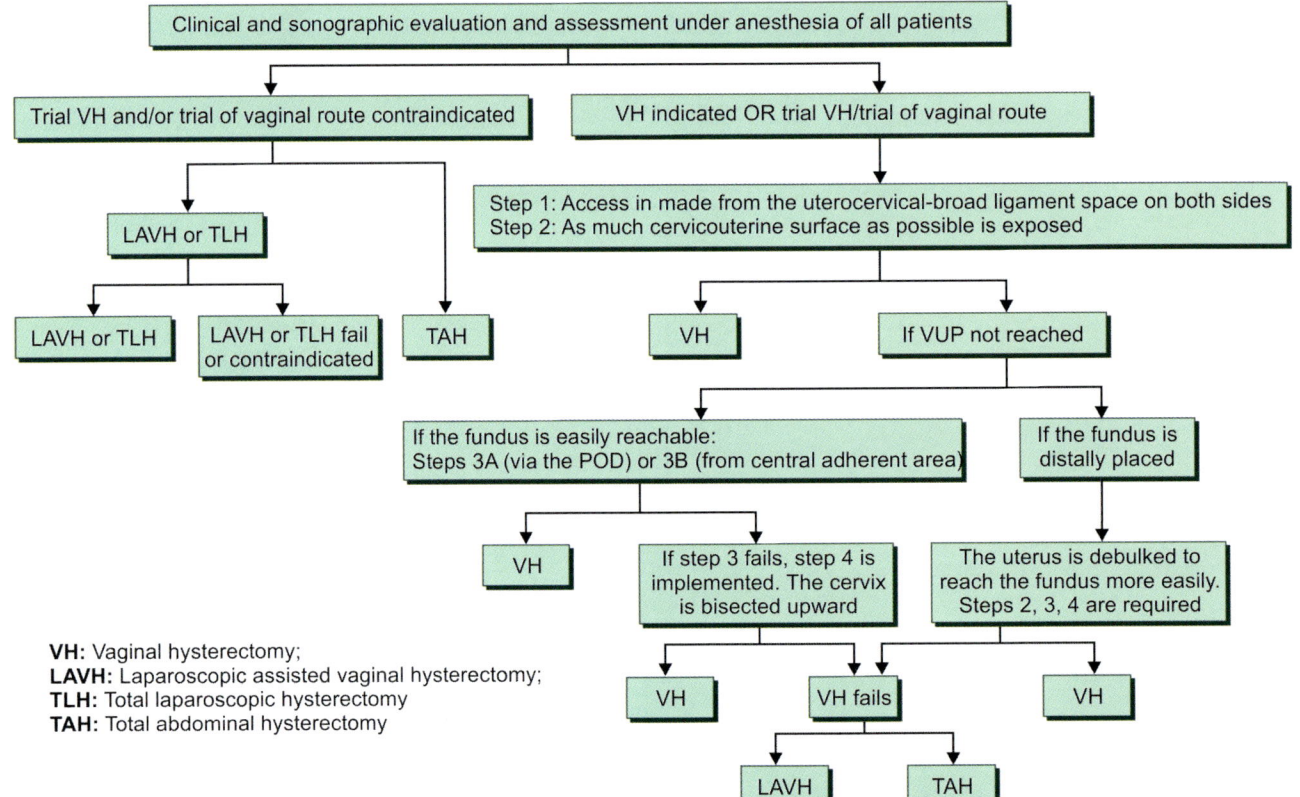

Flow chart 1: Accessing vesicouterine peritoneum (VUP) in women with two or more caesarean deliveries in past, with or without "trial VH and/or trial vaginal route."[4]

VH: Vaginal hysterectomy;
LAVH: Laparoscopic assisted vaginal hysterectomy;
TLH: Total laparoscopic hysterectomy
TAH: Total abdominal hysterectomy

(VH: Vaginal hysterectomy; LAVH: Laparoscopically-assisted vaginal hysterectomy; TLH: Total laparoscopic hysterectomy; TAH: Total abdominal hysterectomy; POD: Pouch of Douglas).

transfusion was not needed. Hospital stay was 2 days with an uneventful speedy recovery (Figs. 1 to 5).

Histopathology showed severe adenomyosis with complex hyperplasia without atypia. Uterus weighed 195 g. No malignancy.

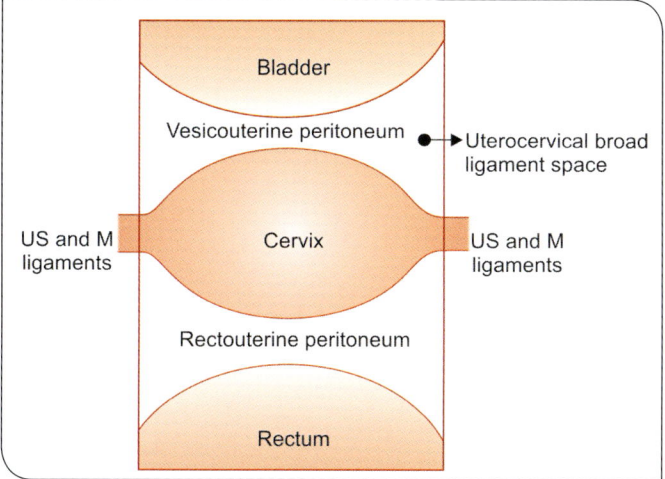

Fig. 1: Distinctly shows the space between bladder and cervix or cervicouterine surface, which is much more under lateral one-fifth of bladder when compared with central three-fifths of bladder.[4]

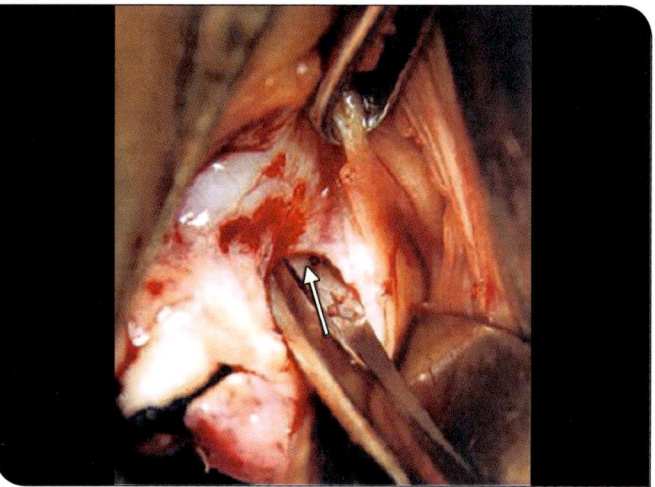

Fig. 2: Entry and access to the uterocervical-broad ligament space. The uterocervical-broad ligament space is widened using scissors while the edge of the anterior vaginal mucosa is held with Allis' forceps and the cervix is pulled with black silk traction sutures.[18]

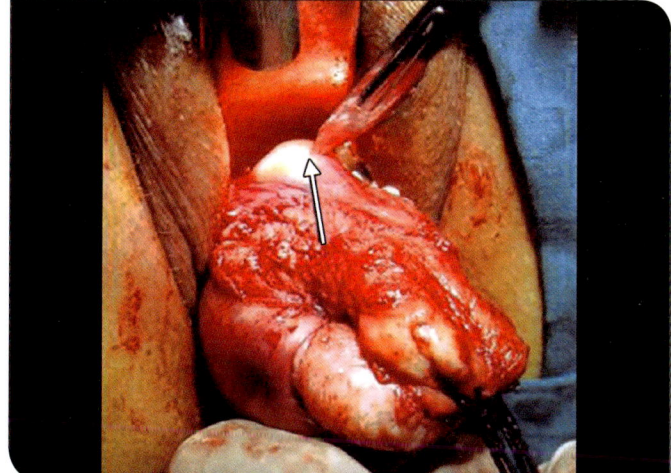

Fig. 3: Access to the vesicouterine peritoneum (VUP) via Step 3Aii. After the uterine vessels are secured and the uterine fundus is brought out of the pouch of Douglas (POD) and pulled as anteriorly as possible, the finger almost reaches the round ligament laterally, then passes through the POD and exits near the right cornual area. Finally, the finger covered by thin peritoneum insinuates itself and appears anteriorly. The peritoneum is then incised to allow the finger to pass through it.[18]

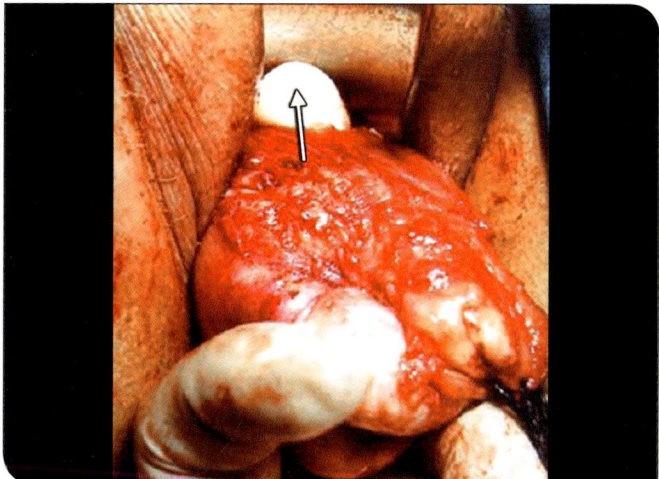

Fig. 4: Access to the vesicouterine peritoneum (VUP) via Step 3Aii. After a finger pushes some of the thin peritoneum anteriorly out of the pouch of Douglas (POD), the peritoneum is incised and the finger emerges. This causes the separation of the bladder from the uterine surface, allowing placement of the bladder retractor.[18]

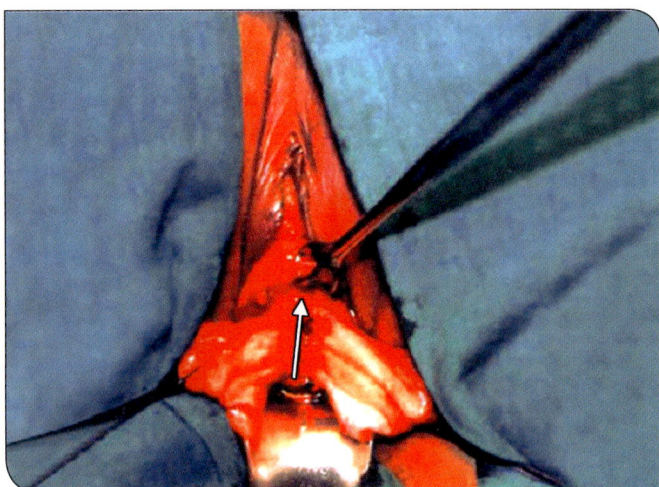

Fig. 5: Cervix bisected to achieve access to the vesicouterine peritoneum (VUP). Slight traction on the bladder with Babcock's forceps brings connecting tissue strands into view for excision and the plane for access.[4]

What inspired: Uterocervical-broad ligament space and H/O three caesarean sections.

LESSON

- Additional step of accessing proximal cornual area and freeing the uterus on one side helped.

REFERENCES

1. Sheth SS, Malpani AN. Vaginal hysterectomy following previous caesarean section. Int J Gynaecol Obstet. 1995;50:165-9.
2. Sheth SS. Vaginal hysterectomy. In: Studd J (Ed). Progress in Obstetrics and Gynecology, Volume 10, 2nd edition. London, UK: Churchill Livingstone; 1993. pp. 317-40.
3. Sheth SS. An approach to vesicouterine peritoneum through a new surgical space. J Gynecol Surg. 1996;12:135-40.
4. Sheth SS. Access to vesicouterine and rectouterine pouches. In: Sheth SS (Ed). Vaginal Hysterectomy, 2nd edition. New Delhi, India: Jaypee Brothers Medical Publishers (P) Ltd; 2014. pp. 31-50.
5. Monaghan JM. A personal communication. 1994.
6. Sizzi O, Paparella P, Bonito C, et al. Laparoscopic assistance after vaginal hysterectomy and unsuccessful access to the ovaries or failed uterine mobilization: changing trends. JSLS. 2004;8(4):339-46.
7. Khung TT. Use of Sheth's uterocervical broad ligament space for vaginal hysterectomy in a patient with history of Caesarean section. Malaysian J Obstet Gynaecol. 1995;4(1-2):39-42.
8. Sheth SS. Vaginal Hysterectomy. Best Pract Res Clin Obstet Gynaecol. 2005;19(3):307-32.
9. Gultekin E, Gultekin OE, Cingillioglu B, et al. The value of frozen section evaluation in the management of borderline ovarian tumors. J Cancer Res Therapeut. 2011;7:416-20.
10. Aarts JW, Nieboer TE, Johnson N, et al. Surgical approach to hysterectomy for benign gynaecological disease. Cochrane Database Syst Rev. 2015;12(8):1-21.
11. Petros P, Ulmsten U. An integral theory on female urinary incontinence. Experimental and clinical considerations. Acta Obstet Gynecol Scand Suppl. 1990;153:7-31.
12. De Leval J. Novel surgical technique for the treatment of female stress urinary incontinence: transobturator vaginal tape inside-out. Euro Urol. 2003;44:724-30.
13. De Leval J, Waltregny D. New surgical technique for treatment of stress urinary incontinence TVT-Obturator: new developments and results. Surg Technol Int. 2005;14:212-21.
14. Sheth SS, Paghdiwalla KP, Hajari AR. Vaginal route: a gynaecological route for much more than hysterectomy. Best Pract Res Clin Obstet Gynaecol. 2011;25(2):115-32.
15. Sheth SS. Newer perspectives. In: Sheth SS (Ed). Vaginal Hysterectomy, 2nd edition. New Delhi, India: Jaypee Brothers Medical Publishers (P) Ltd; 2014. pp. 225-34.
16. Pelosi MA II, Pelosi MA III. Uterine debulking at vaginal hysterectomy. In: Sheth SS (Ed). Vaginal Hysterectomy, 2nd edition. New Delhi, India: Jaypee Brothers Medical Publishers (P) Ltd; 2014. pp. 90-109.
17. Pelosi MA, Pelosi MA III. A comprehensive approach to morcellation of the large uterus. Contemp Obstet Gynecol. 1997;42:106-25.
18. Sheth SS. Vaginal hysterectomy in women with a history of 2 or more caesarean deliveries. Int J Gynecol Obstet. 2013;122:70-4.
19. Sheth SS. Vaginal or abdominal hysterectomy? In: Sheth SS (Ed). Vaginal Hysterectomy, 2nd edition. New Delhi, India: Jaypee Brothers Medical Publishers (P) Ltd; 2014. pp. 273-93.
20. Zanagnolo V, Magrina JF. Vaginal hysterectomy for carcinoma of the endometrium. In: Sheth SS (Ed). Vaginal Hysterectomy, 2nd edition. New Delhi, India: Jaypee Brothers Medical Publishers (P) Ltd; 2014. pp. 216-24.
21. Sheth SS. Adnexectomy for benign pathology at vaginal hysterectomy without laparoscopic assistance. Br J Obstet Gynecol. 2002;109:1401-5.
22. Sheth SS. Adnexal pathology at vaginal hysterectomy. In: Sheth SS (Ed). Vaginal Hysterectomy, 2nd edition. New Delhi, India: Jaypee Brothers Medical Publishers (P) Ltd; 2014. pp. 150-62.
23. Sheth SS. Vaginal hysterectomy as primary route for morbidly obese women. Acta Obstet Gynecol. 2010;89:971-4.
24. Rafii A, Samain E, Levardon M, et al. Vaginal hysterectomy for benign disorders in obese women: a prospective study. Br J Obstet Gynecol. 2005;112:223-7.
25. Lean ME. Prognosis in obesity. BMJ. 2005;330:1339-40.
26. Liston WA, Alexander C. Operating on the obese woman. In: Hillard T (Ed). The Yearbook of Obstetrics and Gynaecology, Volume 12. London, UK: RCOG Press; 2008. pp. 206-9.

27. Kwon JS, Tinker A, Pansegrau G, et al. Prophylactic salpingectomy and delayed oophorectomy as an alternative for BRCA mutation carriers. Obstet Gynecol. 2013;121:14-24.
28. Sheth SS. Vaginal dimple--a sign of ovarian endometriosis. J Obstet Gynecol. 1991;11:292.
29. Sheth SS. The scope of vaginal hysterectomy. Eur J Obstet Gynecol Rep Bio. 2004;115:224-31.
30. Sheth SS, Paghdiwalla K. Do we need the laparoscopic route? J Obstet Gynaecol India. 2001;51:25-30.
31. Sheth SS. A surgical window to access the obliterated posterior cul-de-sac at vaginal hysterectomy. Int J Gynecol Obstet. 2009;107:244-7.
32. Sheth SS. Results of treatment of rupture of the uterus by suturing. J Obstet Gynaec Brit Cwlth. 1968;75:55-8.
33. Sheth SS. Suturing of the tear as treatment in uterine rupture. Am J Obstet Gynecol. 1969;105:440-3.
34. Sheth SS. Vaginal hysterectomy following earlier ruptured uterus and caesarean sections. J Gynecol Surg. 1998;14:185-9.
35. Kovac SR, Cruiskshank SH, Retto HF. Laparoscopy-assisted vaginal hysterectomy. J Gynecol Surg. 1990;6:185-92.
36. Coulam CB, Pratt JH. Vaginal hysterectomy. Is previous pelvic operation a contraindication? Am J Obstet Gynecol. 1973;116:252-60.
37. Hoffman MS, Jaeger M. A new method for gaining entry into the scarred anterior cul-de-sac during transvaginal hysterectomy. Am J Obstet Gynecol. 1990;162(5):1269-70.
38. Sheth SS. Observations from a FIGO Past President on vaginal hysterectomy and related surgery by the vaginal route. Int J Gynecol Obstet. 2016;135:1-4.

CASE 24: VH IN HEAVY CIGARETTE SMOKER WITH H/O TWO CLASSICAL CAESAREAN SECTIONS VIA MIDLINE VERTICAL LAPAROTOMY

Name: Mrs. CS
Age: 51 years
Parity: 2 FT C/S via vertical abdominal incision.
Indication for surgery: Recurrent postmenopause bleeding.
Medical/surgical comorbidity: Smoker half pack per day, umbilical hernia repair.
Operative time: 2 hours (inclusive of cystoscopy).
Hemoglobin pre- and postoperative: 12.7 g/dL, 10.1 g/dL.
Recovery course: Day 1 discharge, rapid activity return, minimal pain.
Pathology report: Uterus 78 g, adenomyosis, leiomyoma (add 10% to uterine weight, specimen sent directly in formalin to pathology; gross weight directly in OR would be 10–15% more).
Preoperative evaluation: Patient 4 years postmenopause with 1 year of persistent vaginal bleeding and thickened endometrium to 0.8 centimeters. Benign hysteroscopic evaluation with biopsy. Patient opted for definitive management. Appropriately counseled as "Trial VH" with possible laparotomy. Premedicated with pyridium for intraoperative cystoscopy. Cervix accessible, uterus mobile, descent very minimal.
What deters/dissuades: Two prior caesareans with vertical abdominal cut, poor descent.
Surgery: Caesarean scar division facilitated by initial bilateral dissection into uterocervical broad ligament spaces.

Lateral pedicle division proceeded uneventfully until round ligaments, at which point significant resistance was met. Centrally anterior peritoneal reflection was not yet accessed. Uterus was bivalved, and this created sufficient exposure to identify and fully enter through anterior peritoneal reflection and then safely clamp, divide, and secure upper pedicles and deliver specimen. Both adnexa were retracted high out of the field of view by atrophic IP ligaments. Brisk bleeding was noted from the peritoneal edge near the left uterosacral ligament pedicle. Gaining exposure to control this bleeder was actually a bit involved due to minimal uterosacral descent and apical retraction of the peritoneal edge, however, eventually an appropriate placed suture achieved hemostasis.

LESSONS

- Vaginal approach, according to statistical evidence, is protective for urinary tract. Anterior scarring from caesarean should not discourage surgeon but actually encourage a vaginal approach provided that the surgeon has comfort with the uterocervical Broad Ligament Space and the preoperative evaluation suggests success is likely.
- A very small uterus with dense central scarring can and often is a more difficult anterior dissection than a large fibroid uterus.
- The American College of Obstetrics and Gynecology guidelines support VH in all feasible patients, including those planned to undergo prophylactic adnexectomy along with their VH. The reason for this is that statistics indicate that: (a) the adnexa are accessible vaginally in the majority of all patients, even those who are postmenopause; and (b) the safety factor of the vaginal approach is such that overall patient morbidity would increase by surgeons routinely abandoning the vagina in these patients in favor of laparoscopy or laparotomy.
- This being said, vaginal surgeons must always be prepared for the possibility of encountering adnexa (either one or both) that are difficult, if not impossible, to access. Such findings at surgery are the result of either pelvic adhesions (the typical issue in a younger patient) or IP ligament atrophy (the typical issue in an elderly postmenopause patient). In such setting-provided the patient in question has no extant adnexal pathology suspected and no elevated risk factors for adnexal malignancy documented in the chart—my personal belief and practice is to leave those inaccessible adnexa in situ and end the operation, accepting the fact that a small minority of my patients may at some point develop a new adnexal pathology requiring further surgery. In this particular case, that is exactly what occurred. One year postoperative the patient presented with pelvic pain and ultrasound revealed a new finding of solid ovarian mass. She underwent laparoscopic BSO, confirming the diagnosis of benign ovarian fibroma.

CASE 25: VH WITH UTERINE DEBULKING PLUS BILATERAL SALPINGECTOMY OF TUBAL REMNANTS AFTER FOUR CAESAREAN SECTIONS AND NO VAGINAL BIRTHS

Name: Mrs. LW
Age: 46 years
Parity: 4 FT C/S, tubal sterilization, no vaginal births.
Indication for surgery: Mass effect, menometrorrhagia.
Medical/surgical comorbidity: None.
Operative time: 2 hours 45 mins (inclusive of cystoscopy and uterosacral suspension).
Hemoglobin pre- and postoperative: 12.7 g/dL, 11.5 g/dL.
Recovery course: Day 1 discharge, rapid return to activity.
Pathology report: Benign oviduct tissue, uterus 404 g, fibroids (add 10% to uterine weight, specimen sent directly in formalin to pathology; gross weight directly in OR would be 10–15% more).
Preoperative evaluation: Benign endometrial biopsy. Mobile uterus, readily accessed cervix. Counseled as "trial VH" with possible laparotomy. Patient thrilled with possibility of avoiding another abdominal cut. Pyridium 3 hours before surgery facilitated cystoscopy at start and end of surgery.

What deters/dissuades: Large uterus, four caesarean deliveries and limited descent.
Surgery: Easy posterior entry. *Uterocervical Broad Ligament Space* accessed bilaterally to facilitate identification central scar plane for sharp dissection. Significant descent after cardinal division allowed completed freeing of bladder from lower segment. After uterine artery division anterior peritoneal reflection identified and entered. Morcellation with intramyometrial coring plus wedge resection proceeded without incident until specimen fully delivered. Both adnexa were easily accessed for ovary inspection and removal of all oviduct remnants.

LESSON

- Number of previous caesareans does not necessarily correlate with extent of adhesive disease or feasibility for vaginal approach. Most important is preoperative evaluation and utilization at surgery of uterocervical broad ligament space.

CASE 26: VH PLUS BILATERAL SALPINGECTOMY AFTER ONE CAESAREAN AND NO VAGINAL BIRTHS

Name: Mrs. AL
Age: 41 years
Parity: 1 FT (full term) caesarean
Indication for surgery: Menorrhagia, dysmenorrhea.
Medical/surgical comorbidity: During early postpartum state patient had massive hemorrhage requiring L uterine artery ablation with 10 units of blood transfusion and two dilatation and curettage (D&C) procedures with subsequent development Asherman's syndrome.
Operative time: 2 hours 15 mins.
Hemoglobin pre- and postoperative: 13 g/dL, 11.1 g/dL.
Recovery course: Day 1 discharge, mild-to-moderate postoperative pain and fatigue resolved after 1 week home convalescence, rapid resumption activity thereafter.
Pathology report: Benign oviducts, uterus 81 g (add 10% to uterine weight, specimen sent directly in formalin to pathology; gross weight directly in OR would be 10–15% more).
Preoperative evaluation: Patient presented on referral requesting hysterectomy for symptom relief. She was counseled to consider alternate treatment options, but she declined, preferring the definitive management offered by hysterectomy. Examination revealed mobile uterus and accessible cervix. Benign endometrial biopsy was obtained.
What deters/dissuades: Limited descent, scarring from prior uterine surgery.
Surgery: Moderate bleeding encountered posteriorly from peritoneal reflection on entry. Sutures to reapproximate edge peritoneum to vaginal cuff achieved hemostasis. Central anterior dissection of very dense caesarean scar facilitated by lateral-to-medial dissection approach, utilizing bilateral uterocervical Broad Ligament Space. Adnexa both easily accessed postuterine delivery.

LESSON

- This case of one caesarean and small uterus should seem comparatively easy compared to previous patient with four caesarean and large uterus. However, degree difficulty intraoperatively was similar, with this surgery involving more blood loss and near same operative time. Again, number prior surgeries is of minimal importance compared to surgeon's preoperative evaluation and comfort with anterior dissection in assessing chance success.

CASE 27: VH WITH UTERINE DEBULKING AFTER SIX MIDLINE VERTICAL LAPAROTOMIES (FIVE CAESAREAN SECTIONS AND ONE ECTOPIC PREGNANCY) IN A MORBIDLY OBESE CIGARETTE SMOKER

Name: Mrs. JY
Age: 50
Parity: G7 P5 (SVD stillbirth 6 lb 13 oz, 5 Caesareans, 1 ectopic)
Indication for surgery: Chronic pain, menorrhagia, anemia, fibroids, suspected adenomyosis
Comorbidities: BMI 43, daily smoker 3 cig/day, 6 prior vertical midline laparotomies
Operative time: 2 hours 20 mins (inclusive of cystoscopy, uterosacral colpo suspension)
Hemoglobin pre- and postoperative: 8.5, 9 (2 units transfused in recovery room)
Pathology: Cervix with chronic inflammation, proliferative endometrium, Uterus 284 grams with numerous intramural fibroids.
Recovery course: Day 1 discharge, minimal pain, rapid activity resumption, foley catheter × 3 days (prophylactic decision made secondary to finding at case end of mild denuded posterior wall bladder mucosa caused by cystoscope trauma)
Preoperative evaluation: Benign endometrial sampling, accessible cervix, uterus seemingly mobile but exam somewhat limited by habitus, physiologic descent with no abdominal dimpling with tenaculum traction on cervix, pelvic ultrasound showed 4 cm cervix without elongation and midline uterus without significant fundal anterior deflection. Counseled as Trial TVH , which patient was enthused to attempt. Pyridium 3 hrs before surgery facilitated cystoscopy at start and end of surgery.
What deters/dissuades: History of 5 caesarean all via midline vertical laparotomy + 1 additional adnexal surgery via vertical midline laparotomy, minimal uterine descent
Surgery: At case start with patient under anesthesia strong traction on cervix again attempted to identify abdominal wall dimpling and none noted. Anteriorly, uterocervical broad Ligament Space easily accessed bilaterally to facilitate identification central scar plane for sharp dissection. Posterior cul de-sac entry easy and routine. Routine progressive descent with division each set lower pedicles allowed completed freeing of bladder from lower segment. After uterine artery division was completed further descent was found to be impeded. Morcellation with bivalve + wedge resection proceeded without incident for majority of specimen. At this point anterior resistance noted and traction on remaining myometrium did show abdominal wall dimpling. Digital exploration identified right ovarian ligament high in pelvis and directed towards sidewall of uterus. Adnexa not palpable and believed adhered to sidewall pelvis. Ovarian ligament pedicle was clamped under tactile guidance, after which retraction allowed for the visual inspection of clamp, confirming proper placement and no incorporation extraneous tissue. Division and securing of this pedicle allowed for delivery of remainder of Right hemi-uterus. Repeat digital exploration revealed Left ovarian ligament and terminal uterine cornua adherent to anterior abdominal wall, however bladder at this point safely free and adhesion plane identified and deemed amenable to blunt division. With this the left ovarian ligament fell into operative field, accessible for easy clamping and division. A normal ovary was inspected. The oviduct was absent, consistent with the patient history.

LESSONS

- Preoperative evaluation for dense uterine to abdominal wall adhesions that preclude Trial TVH include:
  a. Speculum assessment of cervix accessibility.
  b. Traction on cervix to assess for both cervix descent and presence of dimpling of abdomen (this step should be repeated in OR at case onset where one can pull more liberally in anesthetized patient).
  c. Bimanual pelvic exam for uterine mobility.
  d. Transvaginal ultrasound to measure cervix length and and evaluate the relationship of bladder to fundus and relationship fundus to abdominal wall.

  It is important to keep in mind that while "a" and "d" are useful in all patients, "b" and "c" may prove unreliable when evaluating the morbidly obese patients:
- Once again this case demonstrates the utility of the uterocervical broad ligament space to dissect around adhesions, and that the number of previous caesareans does not necessarily correlate with extent of adhesive disease present in the pelvis

- Good descent early on does not guarantee successful completion of the case. Surgeons must know when to abort. With this particular case it was fortunate that abdominal conversion was not required. Had abdominal wall adhesions been identified prior to surgery a trial of Total Vaginal Hysterectomy would likely not have been offered. At the time the adhesions were identified the case was near completed and nonetheless we were prepared to convert the operation. Fortunately, operative exposure and surgeon experience were sufficient to confirm a safe bladder and a tactile adhesion plane amenable to safe division albeit "blind" (in female pelvic anatomy, the surgeon's fingers are often more trustworthy than the eyes at identifying structures)
- As the cystoscopy issue in this case demonstrates, it is critical when operating on smokers not to forget that tissue tends to be friable and poor wound healing is a significant risk. An extra gentle approach to tissue handing, and extra lubrication of scope equipment is helpful in such patients.

Section 2B: VAGINAL HYSTERECTOMY WITH HISTORY OF UTERINE SURGERY IN PAST

CASES

Dr Seth Finkelstein

Case 28: VH in Nullipara with H/O Abdominal Myomectomy
Case 29: VH Plus Salpingectomy in Primipara with H/O Abdominal Myomectomy and Recurrent Large Fibroids

CASE 28: VH IN NULLIPARA WITH H/O ABDOMINAL MYOMECTOMY

Name: Mrs. YJ
Age: 41 years
Parity: 0
Indication for surgery: Menorrhagia, fibroids.
Medical/surgical comorbidity: Abdominal myomectomy 2008 via Maylard incision (549 g myomas removed), 20-year smoker 2–3 cigarettes/day.
Operative time: 1 hour 45 min (inclusive of *cystoscopy* and *uterosacral colposuspension*)
Hemoglobin pre- and postoperative: 12.5 g/dL, no postoperative complete blood count (CBC) due to minimal blood loss.
Recovery course: Day 1 discharge, minimal pain, rapid activity resumption.
Pathology report: Benign right oviduct. Uterus 123 g, fibroids (add 10% to uterine weight, specimen sent directly in formalin to pathology; gross weight directly in OR would be 10–15% more).
Preoperative evaluation: Longstanding patient, earlier myomectomy performed by same surgeon. Presented complaining that she thought her fibroids had returned. After years relief she was again having very heavy menses with clots and dysmenorrhea. She reported having opted against pursuing fertility and that what she wanted at this time was definitive management with hysterectomy.

Examination finding of readily accessed cervix, mobile slight enlarged uterus. Endometrial biopsy was benign.
What deters/dissuades: Concern for scar tissue from prior myomectomy, nulliparity/limited descent.
Surgery: Dense central scarring to bladder present. Left adnexa scarred out of operative view. Right ovary visualized but oviduct involved in scar tissue with ovary and IP (infundibulopelvic) ligament, but sufficiently accessible for sharp adhesiolysis and salpingectomy.

Surgery proceeded methodically and relatively easy with minimal blood loss. Bilateral sharp dissection into *Uterocervical Broad Ligament Spaces* facilitated identification of central scar plane with bladder, thus allowing sharp adhesion release and entry to vesicouterine space (VUS). With each set of pedicles division further uterine descent was obtained, allowing anterior dissection to be continually revisited to advance apical dissection below bladder until entry through anterior peritoneal reflection achieved.

LESSONS

- Risks to urinary tract from scar tissue are dealt with maximum safety and ease with a vaginal approach (abdominal or laparoscopic approaches are riskier) by utilizing the Broad Ligament Space to identify adhesion plane.
- Methodical lateral to medial progression as one advances apically through VUS is the key to success, and in this particular case transformed an extremely difficult operation into a relatively easy one for surgeon and patient.

CASE 29: VH PLUS SALPINGECTOMY IN PRIMIPARA WITH H/O ABDOMINAL MYOMECTOMY AND RECURRENT LARGE FIBROIDS

Name: Mrs. HNM
Age: 51 years
Parity: 1-term spontaneous vaginal delivery (SVD), 1 stillborn SVD 2nd trimester.
Indication for surgery: Dysmenorrhea, menorrhagia, anemia.
Medical/surgical comorbidity: Previous abdominal myomectomy via transverse incision.
Operative time: 3 hours (inclusive of cystoscopy and uterosacral colposuspension).
Hemoglobin pre- and postoperative: 11 g/dL, 9.3 g/dL
Recovery course: Discharge day 1, return to full activity within 1 week.
Pathology report: 443 g, leiomyoma (add 10% to uterine weight, specimen sent directly in formalin to pathology; gross weight directly in OR would be 10–15% more).
Preoperative evaluation: Cervix descent with traction to 1 cm from hymen. Mobile uterus. Hemoglobin 7 g/dL from menorrhagia has increased to 11 g/dL during the month prior to surgery through diet and supplements. Benign endometrial biopsy obtained. Patient after counseling opted for "trial VH".
What deters: Uterine bulk, previous myomectomy.
Surgery: Initial anterior dissection into Uterocervical Broad Ligament Space bilaterally facilitated identification of safe central dissection plane into VUS. Sharp posterior peritoneal entry and division of uterosacral pedicles followed, obtaining descent that allowed further apical entry laterally into Broad Ligament and then centrally under bladder. Stepwise progression in like manner until uterine artery division completed and anterior peritoneum entered. Morcellation techniques of coring and wedge facilitated uterine descent. Bowel adhesions to posterior uterine wall were encountered and sharply divided. After the uterus was completely delivered the right adnexa was noted to be encased in adhesions but the ovary was identified visually and found to be otherwise normal. Left adnexa were readily accessible for salpingectomy and inspection of ovary.

LESSONS

- Myomectomy, even in combination with a large uterus, does not contraindicate "trial VH" in the setting of an otherwise favorable preoperative examination.
- Safe anterior dissection in setting of previous surgery is facilitated by familiarity with broad ligament space. Any bleeding encountered during this lateral dissection is likely to be from cervical descending branch of uterine artery and will be promptly secured upon division of cardinal ligament pedicle.
- Uterine adhesions to bowel that do not significantly impair its descent can be readily dealt with from a vaginal approach using sharp dissection.
- Adnexal access vaginally is the norm in a reproductive age of female, regardless of uterine size. If adnexa are not accessible in such patients the cause is nearly always adhesions. In the elderly, inaccessible adnexa is a more frequent occurrence (1/3 to 1/2 cases) secondary to the added factor of postmenopause atrophy of IP ligaments.

Section 3

VAGINAL HYSTERECTOMY WITH ADNEXAL PATHOLOGY

"In the presence of trouble, some people grow wings; others buy crutches."
—Harold W Ruopp

CASES

Dr Shirish S Sheth

Introduction
Case 30: VH with BSO for Large Bilateral Hydrosalpinx
Case 31: VH with Left Salpingo-oophorectomy for Ovarian Endometrial Cyst in Morbidly Obese with Past History of Two Caesarean Sections
Case 32: VH with BSO for Left Ovarian Endometrial Cyst and Right Ovarian Teratoma with H/O Two Caesarean Sections
Case 33: VH with BSO for Bilateral Ovarian Endometrial Cysts with Positive "Dimple Sign"
Case 34: VH with BSO for a Solid Ovarian Tumor
Case 35: VH with BSO for ?Endometrial Polyp with an Ovarian Solid Tumor
Case 36: VH with BSO followed by Laparotomy for Ovarian Cyst (Failed "Trial Vaginal Route" because of Ovarian "CA")
Case 37: VH with BSO and Right Broad Ligament Myomectomy for Right Broad Ligament Fibroid (BLF)
Case 38: VH with BSO for Twisted Left Ovarian Cyst

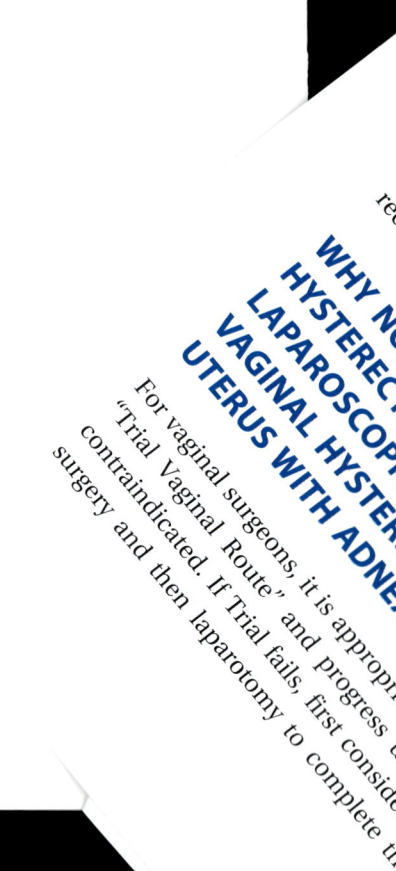

Section 3

VAGINAL HYSTERECTOMY WITH ADNEXAL PATHOLOGY

"In the presence of trouble, some people grow wings; others buy crutches."
—Harold W Ruopp

CASES

Dr Shirish S Sheth

Introduction
Case 30: VH with BSO for Large Bilateral Hydrosalpinx
Case 31: VH with Left Salpingo-oophorectomy for Ovarian Endometrial Cyst in Morbidly Obese with Past History of Two Caesarean Sections
Case 32: VH with BSO for Left Ovarian Endometrial Cyst and Right Ovarian Teratoma with H/O Two Caesarean Sections
Case 33: VH with BSO for Bilateral Ovarian Endometrial Cysts with Positive "Dimple Sign"
Case 34: VH with BSO for a Solid Ovarian Tumor
Case 35: VH with BSO for ?Endometrial Polyp with an Ovarian Solid Tumor
Case 36: VH with BSO followed by Laparotomy for Ovarian Cyst (Failed "Trial Vaginal Route" because of Ovarian "CA")
Case 37: VH with BSO and Right Broad Ligament Myomectomy for Right Broad Ligament Fibroid (BLF)
Case 38: VH with BSO for Twisted Left Ovarian Cyst

INTRODUCTION

For salpingo-oophorectomy at vaginal hysterectomy (VH), cutting and ligating round ligament separately and distally is a "MUST" and that alone facilitates and paves the way to clamp infundibulopelvic ligament (IPL).[1,2] Just as at abdominal hysterectomy (AH), the round ligament is cut separately and as laterally as possible to create a space and apply a clamp to the IPL for salpingo-oophorectomy; the same principle needs to be applied when salpingo-oophorectomy is attempted vaginally, and this step will pave the way to access the IPL. In fact there is hardly any room for the application of two clamps.[1-5]

Crux lies in separating out the round ligament and utilizing the separation for a master step of clamping IPL. Thus it is done in two steps: (1) round ligament to be cut separately and secured and (2) applying clamp on freely available IPL.[2,5-7]

A specially devised clamp[2] with a curve of 2 cm, beginning 1 cm from the tip, Sheth adnexa clamp facilitates and accommodates the IPL, which is transfixed and doubly secured with a No. 1 gauge polyglactin suture or 1/0 Vicryl suture. The ureter is to be safe guarded and it is important to keep that in mind and place the ovarian clamp as medial as possible on the IPL but well beyond ovarian tissue. After completion, it is essential to ensure that there is no raw area distal or lateral to the sutures on IPL that can bleed later.[5,6]

If a salpingo-oophorectomy appears difficult or risky because ovaries are distally placed or an inaccessible IPL, one can reluctantly compromise by performing a simple oophorectomy by clamping, cutting and suturing the mesoovarium.

Debulking of large-sized uterus, removable vaginally, should never contraindicate concomitant oophorectomy/salpingo-oophorectomy at VH as ovarian removal comes into action only after fundus has descended or is just out like in normal size uteri.

Larger uterus means apparently tube and ovaries are distally placed. However, eventually as the fundus descends, tube and ovary have to descend along with the uterus. They are lateral wings or uterine arms and come proximal to the surgeon and become accessible. Therefore, largesized uterus needing debulking should not dissuade performing salpingo-oophorectomy at VH.

Salpingo-oophorectomy is done as usual for mobile, benign adnexal pathology, hydrosalpinx and/or ovarian cyst, but without adhesions, concomitantly at VH, if required after debulking is done and hysterectomy is close to its completion. In other words, to complete debulking and perform hysterectomy with salpingo-oophorectomy. It is preferable to excise all the lateral connections on normal adnexal side. Then after, traction on the uterus helps to cut round ligament distally and access IPL of the pathological side and perform salpingo-oophorectomy. This is followed by salpingo-oophorectomy of contralateral normal adnexal side.[5-8] Before this, if required, vascular small part of broad ligament is occluded to avoid bleeding.

If after massive debulking, access is still difficult, uterus is bisected into two halves to push one half deep inside and deal with tube and ovary of the remaining half of the uterus. Bisected or hemihysterectomized uterus is given gentle traction from medial so as to cut round ligament as laterally as possible. After cutting round ligament laterally, IPL is easily accessed (see salpingo-oophorectomy at VH) to complete salpingo-oophorectomy on one side. This is followed by bringing out contralateral bisected or hemi-hysterectomized debulked uterus and similarly complete the contralateral salpingo-oophorectomy. In fact, total bisection, if done, makes salpingo-oophorectomy easier and helps the operator. Indeed it is an inspiration for young colleagues besides sparing woman from 4 to 5 through and through cuts on the abdominal wall or a greater invasive procedure of opening abdomen.

Hydrosalpinx can be easily punctured and debulked but intact is more satisfying to the operating surgeon, patient plus onlookers and relatives. In fact, if without adhesions or after required adhesiolysis, it is satisfying to deal with benign pathological intact hydrosalpinx and/or intact ovarian cyst.

To debulk, an ovarian cyst can be aspirated. Debulking cyst is easy with a 16 number needle or Veere's needle which is connected to a suction apparatus. However, before inserting the needle into the cyst, all-round area must be safe guarded by an isolation plastic or towel, have head high position and give suprapubic pressure, if required. One may see that contents of the cyst at the most may wet only the isolation sheet and not healthy tissues. Prerequisites are:
- Almost definitively benign pathological adnexa
- Facility for histopathology (HP) frozen study
- Isolation sheet
- Experience of concomitant salpingo-oophorectomy and/or salpingo-oophorectomy of pathological adnexa at VH
- Availability of laparoscopic or laparotomy assistance (Trial Vaginal Route).

Thus, hydrosalpinx and/or ovarian cyst unilateral or bilateral can be easily dealt at VH without the help of a laparoscope.[5-8]

ADHESIONS

Having reached near adnexa during hysterectomy, one attempts to have a clean operative field for salpingo-oophorectomy. If adnexal pathology is with adhesions, for such adhesions, it is usually possible to do gentle adhesiolysis with fingers. Essence is to carefully press healthy surface of tube and/or ovary with finger(s) and take it away from the unhealthy tissue and separate out or push away the unhealthy adherent portion. Tip of finger(s) easily insinuates between the healthy and unhealthy portion of tube and/or ovary and pushes away the unhealthy adherent tissue from the healthy tissue. This often paves the way to hold partially freed ovary and/or tube with Babcock and free it more with scissors. Scissor and finger will do the required adhesiolysis. Adhesions with bowel and/or omentum are easily seen and lysed by holding the intestine/colon gently with Babcock. Small blood vessels are secured to ensure hemostasis. This provides space for further adhesiolysis to free entire tube and/or ovary.[6,8]

PROPHYLACTIC SALPINGECTOMY

What is required is clamping mesosalpinx below the tube and excise the entire tube. Utero-ovarian ligament, ovary and round ligament remain "in situ" as usual after hysterectomy. Salpingectomy without oophorectomy may affect ovarian circulation. However, current literature recommends additional or otherwise at least prophylactic salpingectomy as ovarian cancer may begin from the fimbrial end of the Fallopian tube and therefore, if prophylactic oophorectomy is to be done, it should be salpingo-oophorectomy and not only oophorectomy.[9,10]

WHY NOT TOTAL LAPAROSCOPIC HYSTERECTOMY OR LAPAROSCOPICALLY-ASSISTED VAGINAL HYSTERECTOMY FOR LARGE UTERUS WITH ADNEXAL PATHOLOGY?

For vaginal surgeons, it is appropriate to take the case as "Trial Vaginal Route" and progress unless that is also contraindicated. If Trial fails, first consider laparoscopic surgery and then laparotomy to complete the required surgery. Usually Trial succeeds and enhances operative skill. Thus benign tubal and/or ovarian pathology can be dealt concomitantly at VH and spare greater invasion through laparoscopic surgery or laparotomy, i.e. abdominal invasion.[5,7] Important is profound interest and enthusiasm to tackle within limits of patient's safety and operator's surgical skill and reach. Usually, VH may not be a problem but adnexectomy can be.

TO LEARN

Without any anxiety to perform concomitant salpingo-oophorectomy for benign adnexal pathology at VH. During early period, choose to deal with MOBILE cyst preferably, not big size though size should not matter:
- Simple serous cyst
- Ovarian dermoid/teratoma
- Hydrosalpinx/hematosalpinx
- Endometriotic ovarian cyst: Cyst less than 3 cm, preferably without adhesions. Here small size should not inspire as what matters is "adhesion free". This cannot be forecast and if anxiety or doubts prevail, diagnostic or evaluatory laparoscopy will be helpful. Usually self-confidence, perseverance and keenness to free the ovary from the adhesions will pay richly. Finger(s) and scissor can easily undo and give free ovary and/or tube to deal with.

Such adhesiolysis, ovarian freeing and salpingo-oophorectomy promote confidence and inspire to undertake more and more of it. After some experience, I draw demarcating line at 5–6 cm or less for endometriotic cysts for concomitant salpingo-oophorectomy at VH and attempt it as "trial vaginal route".[7] Beyond 6 cm endometriotic cyst, I take laparoscopic help to free it, perform salpingo-oophorectomy and have laparoscopically-assisted vaginal hysterectomy (LAVH) or have total laparoscopic hysterectomy (TAH). This can vary. Endometriosis of ovary—endometrial cyst of even 3 cm can make VH fail in contrast to even 15 cm serous or dermoid cyst. For nonadherent, nonendometriotic cyst there is no limit for the size, as long as it is benign and can be debulked.

EXCLUDE MALIGNANCY

If facility for frozen HP study is not available and/or there is suspicion or even an iota of doubt about malignancy, vaginal route should be ruled out. Besides this, there can never be 100% guarantee about distinctly benign looking ovarian mass being 100% benign as very uncommonly paraffin HP later, can give an unpleasant surprise or shock. If so, laparotomy becomes mandatory for the omentectomy and lymph node removal, as required. It is wiser and safer to be liberal in asking for frozen HP study rather than getting stumped by paraffin HP study after few days showing malignancy and forcing unexpected and disturbing treatment.

If frozen HP of ovary or tube reports malignancy or suspicion, it is desirable to terminate the vaginal surgery and switch over to opening the abdomen by vertical suprapubic incision and do all that is necessary.[6,8] For contralateral normal ovary, operator can complete that salpingooophorectomy vaginally and then close or do that salpingo-oophorectomy abdominally. Peritoneal lavage fluid is collected for cytological study.

WHY LAPAROTOMY?

Because required surgery cannot be done vaginally, as there is need for:
- Omentectomy
- Inspection of pelvic lymph nodes as well as paraaortic lymph nodes and to perform lymphadenectomy, as required
- Inspection of the liver
- A peritoneal wash for cytology.

ROLE OF SONOGRAPHY-N-SONOLOGIST

Preoperative diagnosis should usually remove the suspicion of malignancy. Sonologist, Dr Darshana Kshirsagar at NM Medical Centre, Mumbai, India has preoperatively reported solid ovarian mass to be (1) ovarian fibroma and thecoma and it turned out to be so. (2) Earlier left solid ovarian tumor diagnosed as malignant by another sonologist, was reported by her as a woman with normal ovaries but with left broad ligament fibroid (BLF). For the latter, I had the pleasure of doing left broad ligament myomectomy concomitantly at VH, sparing abdominal access and confirming the same. Those reported as not benign or likely to be malignant have turned out so. In the presented material, most and not all sonographies are done by her.[6,7]

Trustworthy sonographic opinion is vital for decision making, particularly for: (1) benign ovarian pathology, (2) uterine volume/size (3) size of ovarian cyst and exclusion of endometriosis in early phase of invasive vaginal surgery. She has often advised repeat sonography soon after menses to avoid corpus luteum. Endometriotic ovarian cyst demands more from the operating surgeon. (4) Have "litigation free" as well as "failure free" mind. Just as in obstetrics, forcep is applied as Trial Forcep in select cases and if it succeeds, delivery is vaginal which is gratifying and if it fails, it was not an obstetrician's mistake or failure but anticipated failure, i.e. land up for caesarean section, which was kept available. Such tension-free mind with "desire-n-keenness" to succeed and progress, promotes one to undertake more and more and advance in the surgical outcome.

What promotes vaginal route:
- Least invasive and best in the interest of the patient
- Reliable sonography findings for decision making
- Back up experience of BSO at VH
- Enthusiasm and zeal
- Start with less difficult ones and gradually progress to more difficult cases.

REFERENCES

1. Sheth SS, Malpani AN. Technique of vaginal oophorectomy during vaginal hysterectomy. J Gynecol Surg. 1994;10:197-202.
2. Sheth SS. The place of oophorectomy at vaginal hysterectomy. Br J Obstet Gynecol. 1991;98:662-6.
3. Sheth SS, Malpani A. Routine prophylactic oophorectomy at the time of vaginal hysterectomy in postmenopausal women. Arch Gynecol Obstet. 1992;251:87-91.
4. Sheth SS. Vaginal hysterectomy. Best Pract Res Clin Obstet Gynaecol. 2005;19(3):307-32.
5. Sheth SS. Concomitant salpingo-oophorectomy at vaginal hysterectomy. In: Sheth SS (Ed). Vaginal Hysterectomy, 2nd edition. New Delhi, India: Jaypee Brothers Medical Publishers (P) Ltd; 2014. pp. 137-49.
6. Sheth SS. Adnexal pathology at vaginal hysterectomy. In: Sheth SS (Ed). Vaginal Hysterectomy, 2nd edition. New Delhi, India: Jaypee Brothers Medical Publishers (P) Ltd; 2014. pp. 150-62.
7. Sheth SS, Paghdiwalla KP, Hajari AR. Vaginal route: A gynaecological route for much more than hysterectomy. Best Pract Res Clin Obstet Gynaecol. 2011;25(2):115-32.
8. Sheth SS. Adnexectomy for benign pathology at vaginal hysterectomy without laparoscopic assistance. Br. J Obstet Gynecol. 2002;109:1401-5.
9. Kwon JS, Tinker A, Pansegrau G, et al. Prophylactic salpingectomy and delayed oophorectomy as an alternative for BRCA mutation carriers. Obstet Gynecol. 2013;121:14-24.
10. Xu X, Desai VB. Hospital variation in the practice of bilateral salpingectomy with ovarian conservation in 2012. Obstet Gynecol. 2016;127(2):297-305.

CASE 30: VH WITH BSO FOR LARGE BILATERAL HYDROSALPINX

Name: Mrs. X
Age: 53 years
Parity: Nullipara
Complains of (C/O): Postmenopausal bleeding for 5 days.
Last menstrual period (LMP): 5 years back.

Not obese with no history of (H/O) hypertension or diabetes. Systemic findings were normal. She had a normal size uterus with restricted mobility and a normal cervix which had physiological descent to attempt VH. Tender, cystic to firm mass in both lateral fornices encroaching on the posterior fornix.

Sonography revealed a normal size uterus with volume 50 cm³ with endometrial thickness (ET) of 4 mm plus bilateral hydrosalpinx (right 6.2 cm × 2 cm and left 7.5 cm × 3.8 cm) with normal ovaries.

Diagnosis: Bilateral hydrosalpinx in a nullipara.
Operation: VH with bilateral salpingo-oophorectomy (BSO).
What deters/dissuades VH: Nulliparity.[1]
Examination under anesthesia (EUA): It confirmed that she was fit for a "trial vaginal route"[2,3] case as VH appeared possible. After the uterines were secured, the uterus was fully bisected into two halves, each with intact upper pedicle including the hydrosalpinx on both sides. VH was straightforward.

The tubes and ovaries were adherent to each other and the surrounding area. Lysis was done to free both the tubes and ovaries. Distant flimsy adhesions around the fundus were carefully separated.

Head high position and gravity with suprapubic pressure helped to deliver and exteriorize the hydrosalpinx. The surgical field was well isolated with a sterile plastic sheet. The large left hydrosalpinx was reduced in size by aspiration. Traction on the left half of the uterus gave easy access to the IPL to perform left salpingo-oophorectomy. This provided ample-free space to complete the contralateral salpingo-oophorectomy with traction on the remaining right half of the uterus in a similar fashion and thus complete the hysterectomy with BSO[4,5] (Figs. 1 and 2). Cut open uterus showed normal endometrium. Both salpingo-oophorectomies included the tubes with hydrosalpinx. In both, the round ligaments were cut as laterally as possible,

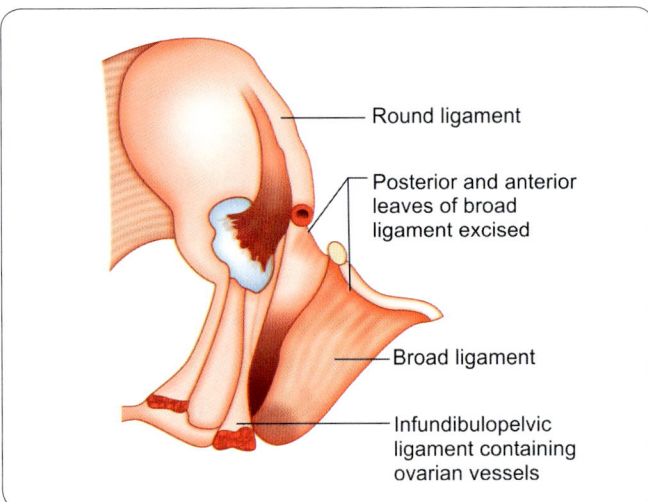

Fig. 1: The round ligament is divided and the retroperitoneal space entered.
Source: Valea FA, Mann WJ. (2014). Open oophorectomy. [online] Available from www.uptodate.com/contents/image?imageKey=OBGYN%2F69337~OBGYN%2F79076~OBGYN%2F58049&topicKey=OBGYN%2F3304&source=see_link&search=open+oophorectomy&utdPopup=true. [Accessed December, 2016]

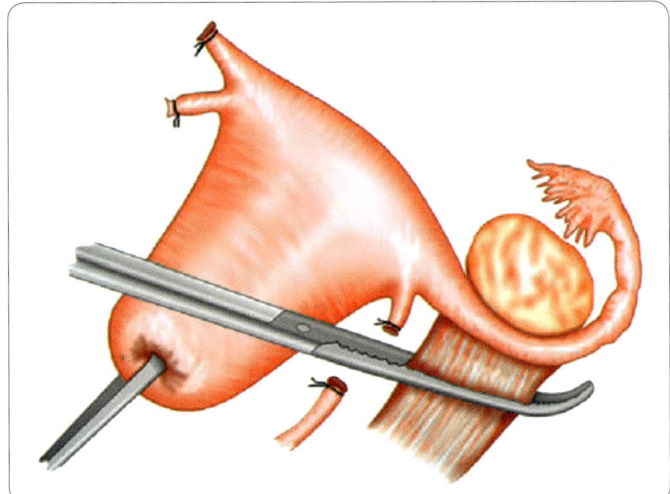

Fig. 2: Round ligament cut distally. A specially designed ovarian clamp is applied to the infundibulopelvic ligament (IPL)
Source: In: Sheth SS (Ed). Vaginal Hysterectomy, 2nd edition. New Delhi, India: Jaypee Brothers Medical Publishers (P) Ltd; 2014. pp. 137-49.

facilitated by traction on the bisected half uterus. Thus, hysterectomy with BSO was completed. Blood transfusion was not needed. Hospital stay was 2 days followed by an uneventful, speedy recovery.

Histopathology showed bilateral hydrosalpinx (6+ cm and 7+ cm size) without malignancy. The uterus, cervix and both ovaries were normal. The uterus weighed 60 g. No malignancy.

What inspired: Experience of concomitant salpingo-oophorectomy at VH and hysterectomies in nullipara.

LESSONS

- Nulliparity should never dissuade VH
- Close to completion of hysterectomy, ample-free space becomes available to deal with adnexal pathology.

CASE 31: VH WITH LEFT SALPINGO-OOPHORECTOMY FOR OVARIAN ENDOMETRIAL CYST IN MORBIDLY OBESE WITH PAST HISTORY OF TWO CAESAREAN SECTIONS

Name: Mrs. X
Age: 38 years
Parity: 2 FTCS
C/O: Heavy and painful menses

Morbidly obese [body mass index (BMI 42)] with no H/O hypertension or diabetes.

Uterus 10+ weeks size, cervix with physiological descent to attempt VH and left ovarian cyst endometriotic. Right and posterior fornices were clear. Sonography confirmed enlarged uterus with 180 cm³ volume and left ovarian endometrial cyst of 6.6 cm × 5.8 cm × 4.3 cm.

Diagnosis: Uterine adenomyosis plus left ovarian endometrial cyst in a morbidly obese patient.

Operation: VH with left salpingo-oophorectomy plus right salpingectomy. Taken as "trial vaginal route" case.

What deters/dissuades: Likely adhesions.

For VH, access to the vesicouterine peritoneum was via the uterocervical-broad ligament space[1,6] (Fig. 1). Pouch of Douglas (POD) was accessed with extra care and hysterectomy completed. Cut open uterus revealed normal endometrium. Left ovary was low down and when held firmly with a Babcock forceps, poured chocolaty material for which a left salpingo-oophorectomy was performed with the help of an ovarian clamp[7,8] (Figs. 2 to 4). Prophylactic right salpingectomy was done.[9] Right healthy ovary preserved as she was very keen to have healthy ovary preserved as she was 38 years old. Hemostasis was checked and vaginal closure done. Blood transfusion was not needed. Hospital stay was 2 days followed by an uneventful speedy recovery.

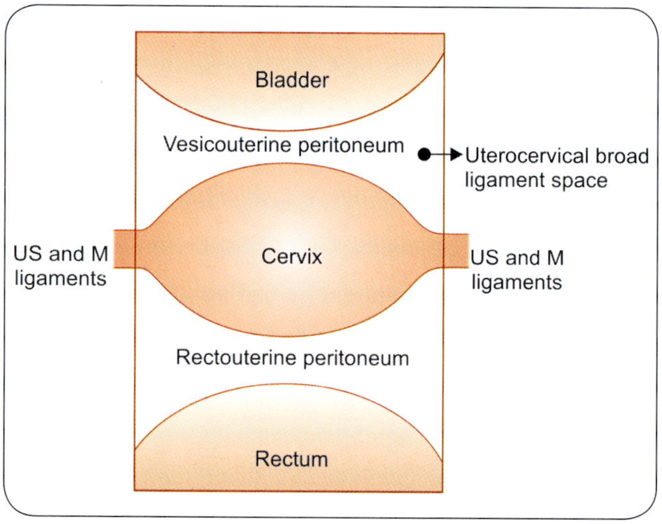

Fig. 1: Distinctly shows the space between bladder and cervix or cervicouterine surface, which is much more under lateral one-fifth of bladder when compared with central three-fifths of bladder
Source: In: Sheth SS (Ed). Vaginal Hysterectomy, 2nd edition. New Delhi, India: Jaypee Brothers Medical Publishers (P) Ltd; 2014. pp. 31-50.

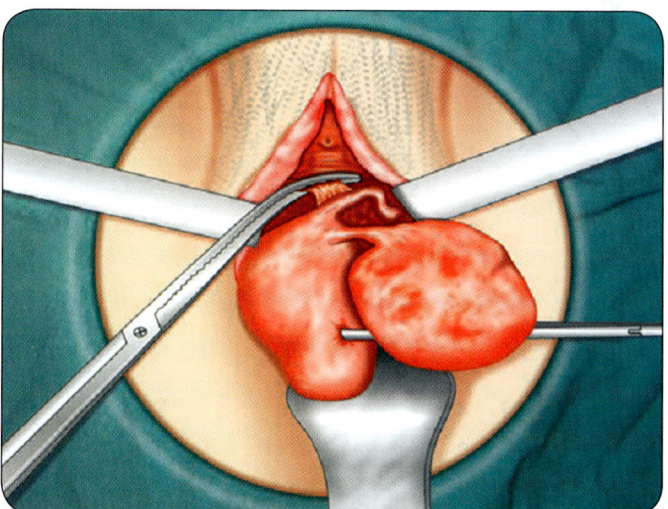

Fig. 2: With all connections on the normal right adnexal side severed, uterus with ovarian cyst with ovarian or adnexal clamp applied on infundibulopelvic ligament (IPL).[4]

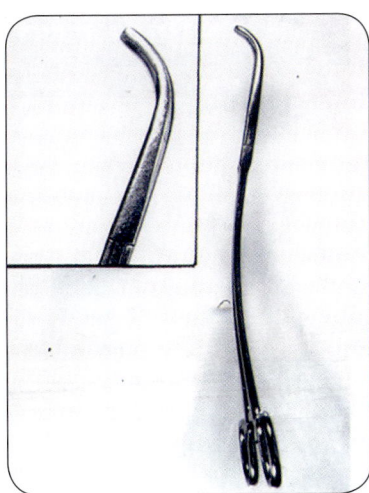

Fig. 3: Specially designed ovarian or Sheth adnexa clamp (Cooper Surgical, USA).[7]

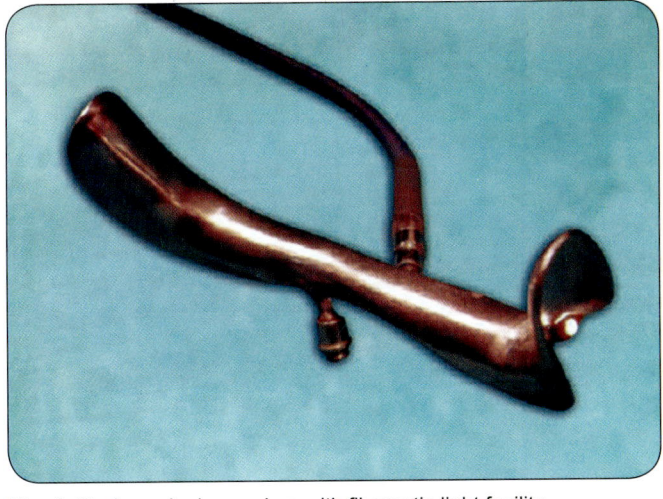

Fig. 4: Sim's vaginal speculum with fiberoptic light facility.
Source: Sheth SS. Fiberoptic light for oophorectomy at vaginal hysterectomy. Obstet Gynec Surv. 1999;54:171-2.

Histopathology showed uterus weighed 213 g with severe adenomyosis. Left ovarian endometriotic cyst and both tubes normal. No evidence of malignancy.

What inspired: VH in a morbidly obese woman[10] with H/O two caesarean sections in past.

LESSONS

- Zeal and endeavor to tackle sizeable endometriotic cyst vaginally
- Two caesarean sections in the past and morbid obesity added flavor.

CASE 32: VH WITH BSO FOR LEFT OVARIAN ENDOMETRIAL CYST AND RIGHT OVARIAN TERATOMA WITH H/O TWO CAESAREAN SECTIONS

Name: Mrs. X
Age: 42 years
Parity: 2 FTCS
LD: 14 years back
C/O: Heavy menses
LMP: 15 days back

The patient was not obese with no H/O hypertension or diabetes. The uterus was 12+ weeks size with fibroids. Cervical descent was favorable to attempt VH but uterine mobility was restricted. A cystic to firm mass in both lateral fornices filling up the posterior fornix were well felt. Sonography showed an enlarged uterus of 300 cm³ volume with a cystic mass of the right ovary, of size 6 cm × 5 cm diagnosed as ovarian teratoma and left adnexal mass with left ovary of size 3 cm × 3 cm as an endometriotic cyst. The tubes were normal.

Diagnosis: Uterine fibroids with right ovarian dermoid and left ovarian endometrial cyst.
Operation: VH with BSO.
What deters/dissuades VH: Bilateral adnexal pathology plus H/O two caesarean sections in the past.

The anterior peritoneum was accessed via the uterocervical-broad ligament space[6] (Fig. 1). The POD was accessed without difficulty as it was occupied by a free, mobile right ovarian cyst. This was followed by hysterectomy, debulking of the uterus being done by enucleation of the fibroids and morcellation of the thick adenomyotic uterine walls. The lateral connections were secured. The right upper pedicle was then severed to make the uterus totally free on the right. The left ovary was freed from flimsy adhesions. The left ovary with a 3 cm × 3 cm cyst was punctured, which oozed out chocolaty material (endometriotic cyst).[4,5] Further traction on the free uterus facilitated hysterectomy with left salpingo-oophorectomy without difficulty, i.e. the uterus with the left tube and ovary including the endometriotic cyst were removed. On naked eye examination, the endometrium was normal in the enlarged adenomyotic uterus with small fibroids. The contralateral right ovary with teratoma and tube were now to be dealt with (Fig. 2).

The right ovary was not visible and needed suprapubic pressure with a head high position, for visualization and access by a Babcock forceps. The area was isolated all around to debulk the cyst 6 cm × 5 cm in size which felt firm to cystic and was mobile. Debulking of the cyst was done by putting a Veress needle and aspirating thick,

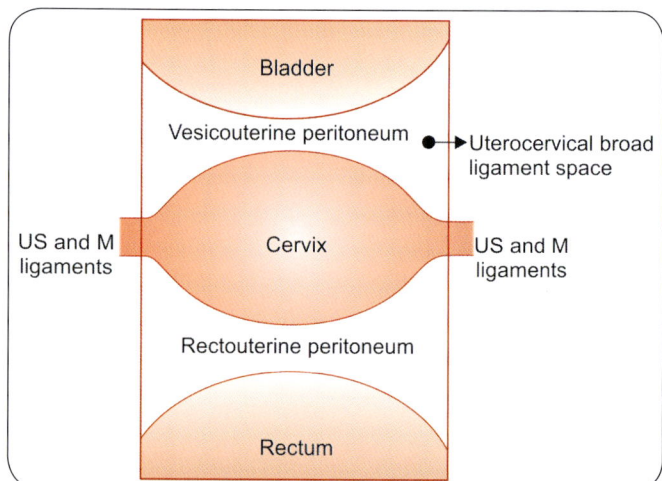

Fig. 1: Distinctly shows the space between bladder and cervix or cervicouterine surface, which is much more under lateral one-fifth of bladder when compared with central three-fifths of bladder.
Source: In: Sheth SS (Ed). Vaginal Hysterectomy, 2nd edition. New Delhi, India: Jaypee Brothers Medical Publishers (P) Ltd; 2014. pp. 31-50.

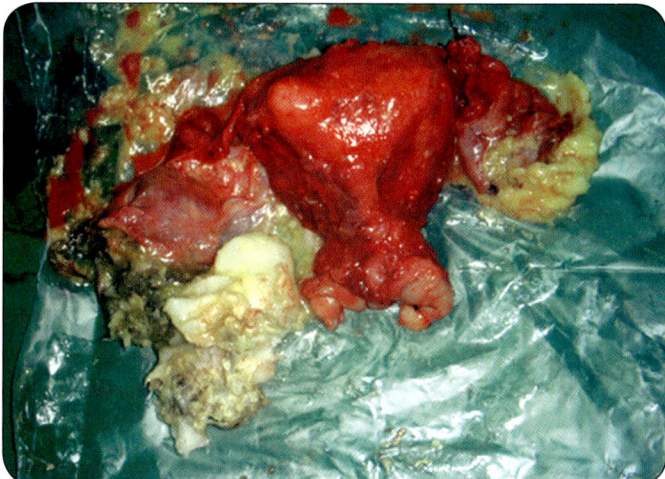

Fig. 2: Dermoid or teratoma on uterine right side and endometriotic cyst on left (entire specimen put on spilled contents from the dermoid cyst).

dirty material which confirmed the diagnosis of ovarian teratoma.[2,4,11-15] The needle was connected to a suction apparatus. There was zero spillage on healthy tissues. Right salpingo-oophorectomy was completed as the patient was not keen to preserve her ovaries. Hemostasis was checked and closure done. Blood transfusion was not needed. Hospital stay was 2 days followed by an uneventful, speedy recovery.

Histopathology study: Uterus weighed 360 g with severe adenomyosis plus small fibroids, right ovarian teratoma and left ovarian endometriosis. No malignancy detected.

What inspired:
- Past experience of endometriotic cystectomy as well as salpingo-oophorectomy at VH
- Benign, mobile right ovarian dermoid added flavor.

LESSONS

- History of two caesarean sections did not change the decision
- Salpingo-oophorectomy for ovarian dermoid cyst was straightforward but left ovarian endometriosis needed extra care.

CASE 33: VH WITH BSO FOR BILATERAL OVARIAN ENDOMETRIAL CYSTS WITH POSITIVE "DIMPLE SIGN"

Name: Mrs. X
Age: 46 years
Parity: 1 FTCS
LD: 20 years back
C/O: Prolonged, heavy and painful menses.
H/O: Laparoscopic surgery twice for ovarian endometriosis.

Normal size uterus with restricted mobility. Cervix: Healthy with physiological descent to attempt VH. Both lateral and posterior fornices with tender firm mass. Clinically presence of the "Dimple sign"[16] showing obliteration of POD because of ovarian endometriosis. Sign was later confirmed under anesthesia.

Sonography: Uterus volume 100 cm^3, right ovary with 2.7 cm × 1.5 cm endometriotic cyst. Right tube normal. Left ovary with 3.1 cm × 1 cm endometriotic cyst plus left tubal hydrosalpinx.
Diagnosis: Bilateral ovarian endometrial cysts.
Operation: VH with BSO.
What deters/dissuades: Positive "Dimple sign".

Anterior peritoneum was accessed with the help of uterocervical-broad ligament space.[6] Access to POD or posterior peritoneum was obtained by separating the soft tissue away from the posterior cervicouterine surface so as to feel firm posterior cervicouterine surface directly and get an access to the peritoneum from the posterior space (Fig.1). Access was realized by pouring of chocolaty material.[17] Escape of chocolaty material or fluid from POD is a good sign—a highly satisfying one.

Uterus was totally bisected from the cervix till fundus to deal with each adnexectomy with the help of traction on hemihysterectomized or half uterus. Tubes and ovaries were densely adherent to the surrounding tissues. Left ovary was smaller than the right because of a H/O two ovarian cystectomies in the past. After adhesiolysis the tubes and ovaries were freed for BSO. Traction on hemihysterectomized uterus felicitated access to each IPL after cutting the round ligament as laterally as possible.[4,5] No endometriotic tissue was seen in the operative field. Hysterectomy with BSO was completed.[3] Cut open uterus showed normal endometrium. Hemostasis was checked and vaginal closure done. Blood transfusion was not needed. Hospital stay was 2 days followed by an uneventful speedy recovery.
Histopathology: It revealed normal uterus, bilateral severe ovarian endometriosis, normal tubes and no malignancy.

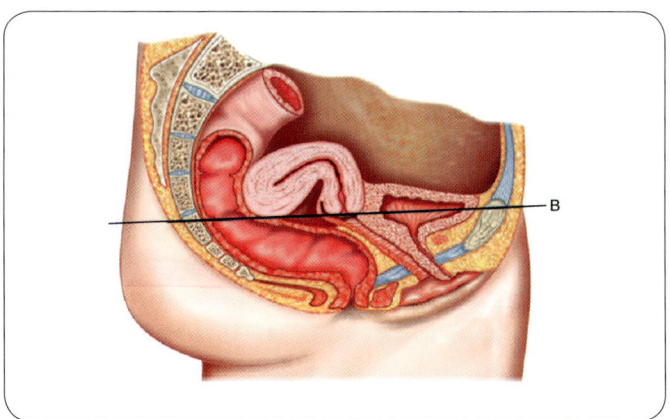

Fig. 1: A marked retroversion with retroflexion creates a space between the uterocervical junction and the B line.
Source: Prepared by surgeon, Dr RD Prabhu, Shimoga, Karnataka, India.[17]

What inspired:
- Experience of dealing with ovarian endometriosis and obliterated POD
- The endometrial cysts were not large
- Taken as "trial vaginal route" case.

LESSONS

- Adhesiolysis gave access to the POD and later freed the tubes and ovaries
- H/O caesarean section in past added flavor.

DISCUSSION

It was noted that there was open space, consistently present in women with a retroverted, retroflexed uterus. It is described as a recto-uterocervical pouch (or posterior uterocervical-broad ligament space), located between the posterior aspects of the uterus and cervix proximally, two leaves of the broad ligament laterally and the rectum posteriorly (Figs. 1 and 2). The posterior of the uterocervical angle forms the apex of this space, its depth depends on the presence or absence of adhesions or mass(es) and the degree of retroflexion of the uterus and the width that of the uterocervical junction, plus about 1 cm on either side between the two leaves of the broad ligament (Fig. 3). When the POD is free, the space extends from a plane joining the posterior uterine body's bulge to the posterior

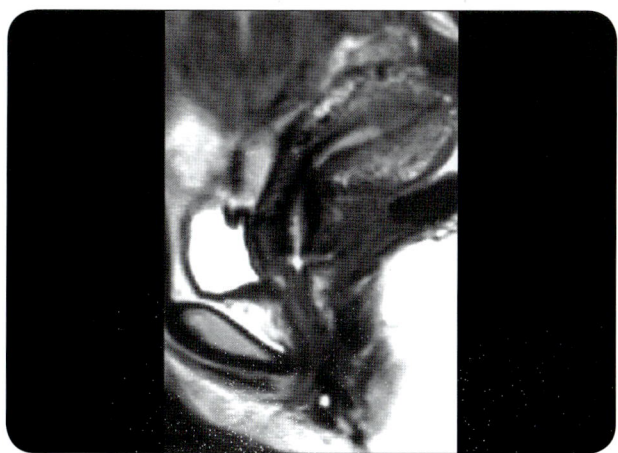

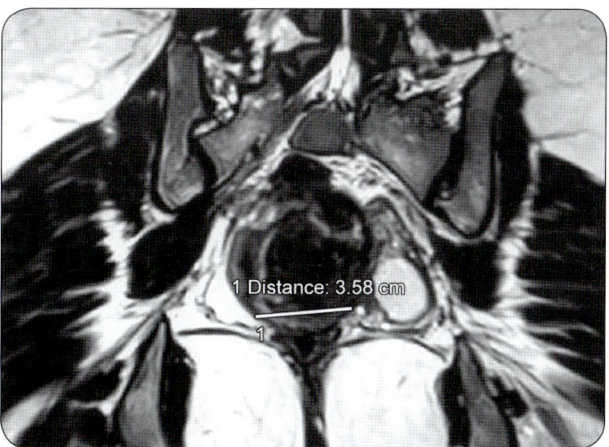

Fig. 2: MRI showing a retroverted and retroflexed uterus as well as the posterior uterocervical-broad ligament space, which measured 1.36 cm vertically and 0.73 cm transversally.
Source: MRI prepared by Dr Nilesh Shah and Dr Manjari Bapat, Mumbai, Maharashtra, India.[1]

Fig. 3: MRI showing the width of the transverse posterior uterocervical-broad ligament space; it is the width of the uterocervical junction, plus 1 cm to the broad ligament on both sides.
Source: MRI prepared by Dr Nilesh Shah and Dr Manjari Bapat, Mumbai, Maharashtra, India.[17]

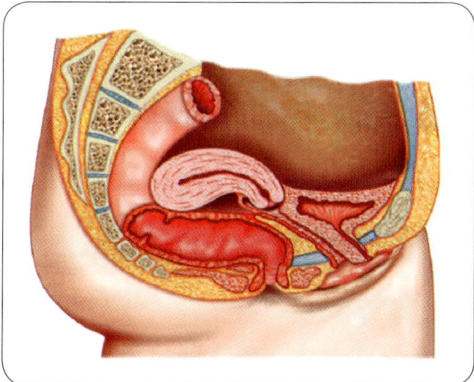

Fig. 4: Adherent mass in the posterior uterocervical-broad ligament space.
Source: Prepared by surgeon, Dr RD Prabhu, Shimoga, Karnataka, India.[17]

bulge of the cervix to the uterocervical angle in front. One can therefore attempt to gain access to the posterior wall of the uterus in most women through this surgical space. Posteriorly the space is continuous with the pelvic peritoneal cavity except when adhesions obstruct it, partly or wholly.

When the retroverted uterus is restored to its normal position, the posterior uterocervical-broad ligament space vanishes. This space can be partly obstructed by an adherent mass (Fig. 4), but its apex almost always remains like a window, large enough for a finger or a small swab on a holder to separate the mass and gain access into the space and from there to other parts of the POD. Once the posterior uterocervical-broad ligament space is completely free of adhesions, the uterus can be grabbed with a pair of Allis' forceps and brought into view. Anteversion creates a similar space on the anterior side of the uterus, and it can also be used as a surgical window to access anterior peritoneal adhesions during LAVH or AH.

Thus the posterior uterocervical-broad ligament space as a surgical window can give entry for the removal of the pathological adnexa vaginally at VH in some women with ovarian endometriosis even when the POD is obstructed or the "Dimple sign" is positive. However, it is not as easy as getting uterocervical-broad ligament space anteriorly to separate the bladder laterally for women with H/O caesarean section in past.

The following points paved the way:
- Making the posterior cervicouterine surface as bare as the anterior uterocervical surface with a finger and a swab on a holder, and/or via extraperitoneal subcervical tunneling
- Securing the uterine vessels, extraperitoneally, if necessary
- Clearing the posterior uterocervical-broad ligament space by first lysing the adhesions below and/or above the uterocervical junction and utilizing it
- Trying to find an access to the peritoneal cavity from the safer and easier, nonpathologic side.

CASE 34: VH WITH BSO FOR A SOLID OVARIAN TUMOR

Name: Mrs. X
Age: 52 years
Parity: 2 FTND (full term normal delivery)
LD: 20 years back
C/O: Spotting per vaginam for 3 months.

Not obese, no H/O hypertension or diabetes. Uterus was 12+ weeks size, freely mobile. Cervix was healthy with restricted cervical descent, less than physiological descent. Fornices were clear except for a firm to solid right adnexal mass.

Sonography: It showed uterus 9.8 cm × 8.5 cm × 7.3 cm, volume 328 cm^3. Endometrial polyp 1 cm, ET 12 mm with right ovarian solid tumor of 4 cm × 2 cm with RI resistance index 0.62. Benign tumor (?Brenner).

Diagnosis: Uterine fibroids plus right ovarian ?Brenner tumor.

Operation: VH with BSO.

What deters/dissuades: Restricted descent of cervix and a solid ovarian tumor.

Started as "trial VH" because of restricted descent of cervix.[2,3] Uterus needed debulking because of fibroids with adenomyosis to complete the hysterectomy.[3] Right ovary showed a firm to hard mass of 3 cm × 2 cm which was carefully excised and remaining healthy right ovary was kept intact. Uterus and right ovarian mass were sent for frozen HP study as the patient was keen to preserve her ovaries, if normal and, if possible. Frozen HP reported no malignancy of uterus as well as ovarian mass. Ovarian mass was reported as benign Brenner tumor of the ovary. In light of the right ovarian tumor, it was preferred to have BSO (age: 52 years).[4,5,7,8] Preoperatively it was discussed and she was counseled that ovaries will be preserved, if healthy and if not, they will be removed. For this she had given her consent. Hemostasis was checked and vaginal closure done. Blood transfusion was not needed. Hospital stay was 2 days followed by an uneventful speedy recovery.

Histopathology report: It showed uterus of 330 g with severe adenomyosis and leiomyomatous. Right ovary showed benign Brenner tumor. Left ovary and both tubes were normal. No evidence of malignancy.

What inspired: Availability of frozen HP study.

LESSON

- Benign solid ovarian tumor dealt with vaginally at VH. Trustworthy sonologist.

CASE 35: VH WITH BSO FOR ?ENDOMETRIAL POLYP WITH AN OVARIAN SOLID TUMOR

Name: Mrs. X
Age: 64 years
Parity: 1 FTND
LD: 32 years back
C/O: Postmenopausal bleeding.
LMP: 15 years back.

The patient was morbidly obese (BMI: 42)[10] with H/O hypertension and no H/O diabetes. She complained of pain in the lower abdomen since 2 months.

The uterus was normal in size with free mobility. A healthy cervix with physiological descent encouraged to attempt VH. There was a firm to solid mass in the left fornix.

Sonographic findings: A normal uterus with a volume of 30 cm³. The ET was 10 mm. The right tube and ovary were normal. The left ovary showed a 5.3 cm × 4 cm solid tumor (Fig. 1) with RI of 0.65 and was reported by experienced sonologist Dr Darshana Kshirsagar, Consultant Radiologist, NM Medical Centre, Mumbai, India as thecoma or fibroma but no malignancy. In other words, it was a benign ovarian tumor. The left tube was normal.

Diagnosis: Benign ovarian fibrothecoma with benign endometrial polyp.

Operation: VH with BSO.

What deters/dissuades: A solid ovarian tumor plus pathological ET 10 mm.

As she could have endometrial "Cancer (CA)", VH with a vaginal cuff of 3–4 cm was performed till the upper pedicles.[3,18,19] The left ovarian mass adherent to the bowel was carefully separated. The right upper uterine connections were severed to free the uterus on the right side, as the adnexal pathology was on the left. Operative field was made safe by an isolation sheet. The left pathological adnexa or upper pedicle was intact, attached to the uterus. The left round ligament was cut distally or as laterally as possible and left salpingo-oophorectomy completed by clamping the IPL, including the INTACT ovarian mass.[4,5] Thus the hysterectomy with left salpingo-oophorectomy was completed. The cut uterus showed a benign looking polyp, with normal looking endometrium. The uterus and left ovarian mass were sent for frozen section HP study. Meanwhile the contralateral normal right tube and ovary were excised by performing right salpingo-oophorectomy and thus hysterectomy with BSO was completed. Frozen section HP report diagnosed benign endometrial polyp with benign ovarian fibrothecoma. No malignancy of endometrium as well as ovary detected. Blood transfusion was not needed. Hospital stay was 2 days, followed by an uneventful, speedy recovery.

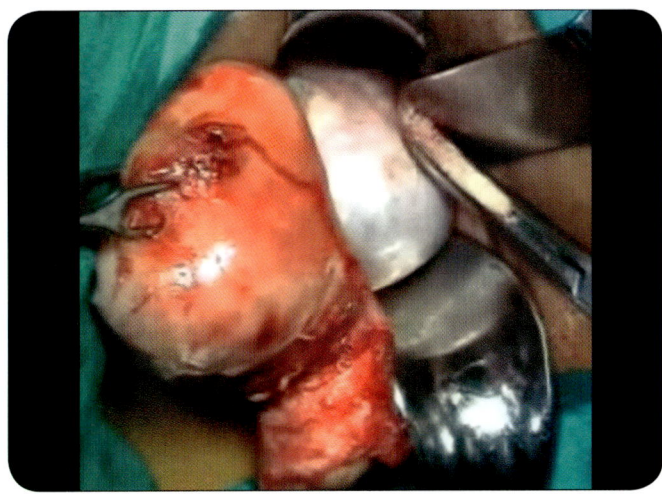

Fig. 1: Left ovarian tumor. All contralateral connections are severed to free the uterus for traction and perform right salpingo-oophorectomy.

Postoperative paraffin HP study reported a uterus of 35 g weight with mild adenomyosis, benign uterine polyp and benign endometrium. The left ovary was confirmed to be a benign fibrothecoma. There was no evidence of malignancy. The right ovary and both tubes were normal.

What inspired:
- A reliable sonography diagnosis of solid ovarian tumor as benign mass (fibroma OR thecoma)
- Experience of concomitant salpingo-oophorectomy for benign adnexal pathology at VH
- If at all, the report of frozen section HP of uterus is malignancy, hopefully it would not have invaded more than half of the myometrial wall. In other words, lymph node removal would have been unnecessary and therefore, VH plus BSO would suffice
- A morbidly obese and hypertensive woman got the advantage of not having her abdomen cut with the resultant morbidity.

LESSON

- With reliable sonography report, vaginal route is comfortably possible, provided frozen HP is available.

What added flavor: Frozen section showing no endometrial "CA".

CASE 36: VH WITH BSO FOLLOWED BY LAPAROTOMY FOR OVARIAN CYST (FAILED "TRIAL VAGINAL ROUTE" BECAUSE OF OVARIAN "CA")

Name: Mrs. X
Age: 48 years
Parity: 3 FTND
LD: 16 years back
C/O: Lower abdominal pain and painful coitus (dyspareunia).

Not obese. No H/O hypertension or diabetes.

Clinically uterus 10 weeks size, freely mobile. Normal cervix with physiological descent to attempt VH. Left fornix had cystic to firm mass encroaching posterior fornix. Right and anterior fornices were clear.

Sonography showed enlarged uterus with 190 cm^3 volume, left ovarian cyst of 8 cm × 4 cm with multiseptation including thick septum and irregular outline without solid area. RI was 0.46. Right tube and ovary were normal.

Diagnosis: Left ovarian tumor.

Operation: VH with BSO → Ovarian adenocarcinoma → Failed "TRIAL vaginal route" → Abdominal omentectomy and lymph nodes removal.

This was discussed at length, including frozen HP, during vaginal surgery. Well-informed consent was taken for "Trial Vaginal Route" case.[2,3] VH was straightforward. After uterines were secured, on reaching both upper pedicles, all lateral connections on the right were cut to make the uterus free on that side. Right tube and ovary were normal. A plastic sheet was spread all over the operative field to avoid contamination. Left ovarian surface appeared normal, shining without excrescences and adhesions. Suprapubic pressure aided by uterine traction exteriorized the left ovarian mass[4,5,11] and cutting round ligament distally. Thus hysterectomy was completed along with left salpingo-oophorectomy including INTACT ovarian mass. Cut open uterus showed normal endometrium. Uterus with left tube and ovary was sent for frozen HP study to find out ovarian pathology. The frozen section analysis should be done by an experienced pathologist and the possible predictive factors affecting a false diagnosis should carefully be taken into consideration.[20] Meanwhile, contralateral right salpingo-oophorectomy was completed. Frozen HP reported ovarian malignancy, well-differentiated adenocarcinoma. After collecting peritoneal and lavage fluid for cytological study, vaginal closure was done and she was put in a position for laparotomy. The abdomen opened by a right paramedian incision. Necessary inspection showed normal findings. Required omentectomy with bilateral pelvic lymphadenectomy was done. Liver, diaphragm, paraaortic and inferior vena caval areas were normal. Fluid from paracolic gutters and peritoneal cavity was collected for cytology and closure done. She had an uneventful postoperative recovery.

Paraffin HP reported, well-differentiated adenocarcinoma of left ovary with normal tubes, right ovary and uterus. Uterus weighed 210 g and showed moderate adenomyosis. Lymph nodes and omentum were negative for malignancy.

She was referred to an oncosurgeon for an opinion before subjecting to chemotherapy. While dealing with adnexal pathology, particularly ovarian it is essential to have extra bit of preoperative counseling, informed consent and keep availability of frozen HP study and laparotomy to spare from untoward aftermath.

What inspired: Trial Vaginal Route but in a wrong case.

LESSONS

- Frozen HP and readiness to switch over to laparotomy
- Taking her as "TRIAL vaginal route" was less disturbing.

CASE 35: VH WITH BSO FOR ?ENDOMETRIAL POLYP WITH AN OVARIAN SOLID TUMOR

Name: Mrs. X
Age: 64 years
Parity: 1 FTND
LD: 32 years back
C/O: Postmenopausal bleeding.
LMP: 15 years back.

The patient was morbidly obese (BMI: 42)[10] with H/O hypertension and no H/O diabetes. She complained of pain in the lower abdomen since 2 months.

The uterus was normal in size with free mobility. A healthy cervix with physiological descent encouraged to attempt VH. There was a firm to solid mass in the left fornix.

Sonographic findings: A normal uterus with a volume of 30 cm³. The ET was 10 mm. The right tube and ovary were normal. The left ovary showed a 5.3 cm × 4 cm solid tumor (Fig. 1) with RI of 0.65 and was reported by experienced sonologist Dr Darshana Kshirsagar, Consultant Radiologist, NM Medical Centre, Mumbai, India as thecoma or fibroma but no malignancy. In other words, it was a benign ovarian tumor. The left tube was normal.

Diagnosis: Benign ovarian fibrothecoma with benign endometrial polyp.
Operation: VH with BSO.
What deters/dissuades: A solid ovarian tumor plus pathological ET 10 mm.

As she could have endometrial "Cancer (CA)", VH with a vaginal cuff of 3–4 cm was performed till the upper pedicles.[3,18,19] The left ovarian mass adherent to the bowel was carefully separated. The right upper uterine connections were severed to free the uterus on the right side, as the adnexal pathology was on the left. Operative field was made safe by an isolation sheet. The left pathological adnexa or upper pedicle was intact, attached to the uterus. The left round ligament was cut distally or as laterally as possible and left salpingo-oophorectomy completed by clamping the IPL, including the INTACT ovarian mass.[4,5] Thus the hysterectomy with left salpingo-oophorectomy was completed. The cut uterus showed a benign looking polyp, with normal looking endometrium. The uterus and left ovarian mass were sent for frozen section HP study. Meanwhile the contralateral normal right tube and ovary were excised by performing right salpingo-oophorectomy and thus hysterectomy with BSO was completed. Frozen section HP report diagnosed benign endometrial polyp

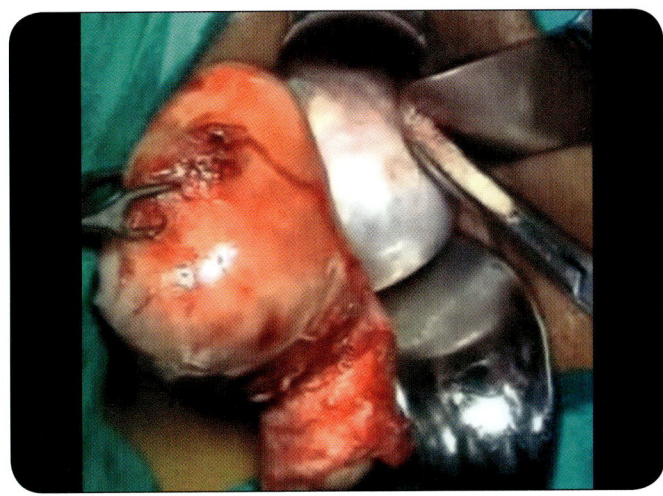

Fig. 1: Left ovarian tumor. All contralateral connections are severed to free the uterus for traction and perform right salpingo-oophorectomy.

with benign ovarian fibrothecoma. No malignancy of endometrium as well as ovary detected. Blood transfusion was not needed. Hospital stay was 2 days, followed by an uneventful, speedy recovery.

Postoperative paraffin HP study reported a uterus of 35 g weight with mild adenomyosis, benign uterine polyp and benign endometrium. The left ovary was confirmed to be a benign fibrothecoma. There was no evidence of malignancy. The right ovary and both tubes were normal.

What inspired:
- A reliable sonography diagnosis of solid ovarian tumor as benign mass (fibroma OR thecoma)
- Experience of concomitant salpingo-oophorectomy for benign adnexal pathology at VH
- If at all, the report of frozen section HP of uterus is malignancy, hopefully it would not have invaded more than half of the myometrial wall. In other words, lymph node removal would have been unnecessary and therefore, VH plus BSO would suffice
- A morbidly obese and hypertensive woman got the advantage of not having her abdomen cut with the resultant morbidity.

LESSON
- With reliable sonography report, vaginal route is comfortably possible, provided frozen HP is available.

What added flavor: Frozen section showing no endometrial "CA".

CASE 36: VH WITH BSO FOLLOWED BY LAPAROTOMY FOR OVARIAN CYST (FAILED "TRIAL VAGINAL ROUTE" BECAUSE OF OVARIAN "CA")

Name: Mrs. X
Age: 48 years
Parity: 3 FTND
LD: 16 years back
C/O: Lower abdominal pain and painful coitus (dyspareunia).

Not obese. No H/O hypertension or diabetes.

Clinically uterus 10 weeks size, freely mobile. Normal cervix with physiological descent to attempt VH. Left fornix had cystic to firm mass encroaching posterior fornix. Right and anterior fornices were clear.

Sonography showed enlarged uterus with 190 cm^3 volume, left ovarian cyst of 8 cm × 4 cm with multiseptation including thick septum and irregular outline without solid area. RI was 0.46. Right tube and ovary were normal.

Diagnosis: Left ovarian tumor.

Operation: VH with BSO → Ovarian adenocarcinoma → Failed "TRIAL vaginal route" → Abdominal omentectomy and lymph nodes removal.

This was discussed at length, including frozen HP, during vaginal surgery. Well-informed consent was taken for "Trial Vaginal Route" case.[2,3] VH was straightforward. After uterines were secured, on reaching both upper pedicles, all lateral connections on the right were cut to make the uterus free on that side. Right tube and ovary were normal. A plastic sheet was spread all over the operative field to avoid contamination. Left ovarian surface appeared normal, shining without excrescences and adhesions. Suprapubic pressure aided by uterine traction exteriorized the left ovarian mass[4,5,11] and cutting round ligament distally. Thus hysterectomy was completed along with left salpingo-oophorectomy including INTACT ovarian mass. Cut open uterus showed normal endometrium. Uterus with left tube and ovary was sent for frozen HP study to find out ovarian pathology. The frozen section analysis should be done by an experienced pathologist and the possible predictive factors affecting a false diagnosis should carefully be taken into consideration.[20] Meanwhile, contralateral right salpingo-oophorectomy was completed. Frozen HP reported ovarian malignancy, well-differentiated adenocarcinoma. After collecting peritoneal and lavage fluid for cytological study, vaginal closure was done and she was put in a position for laparotomy. The abdomen opened by a right paramedian incision. Necessary inspection showed normal findings. Required omentectomy with bilateral pelvic lymphadenectomy was done. Liver, diaphragm, paraaortic and inferior vena caval areas were normal. Fluid from paracolic gutters and peritoneal cavity was collected for cytology and closure done. She had an uneventful postoperative recovery.

Paraffin HP reported, well-differentiated adenocarcinoma of left ovary with normal tubes, right ovary and uterus. Uterus weighed 210 g and showed moderate adenomyosis. Lymph nodes and omentum were negative for malignancy.

She was referred to an oncosurgeon for an opinion before subjecting to chemotherapy. While dealing with adnexal pathology, particularly ovarian it is essential to have extra bit of preoperative counseling, informed consent and keep availability of frozen HP study and laparotomy to spare from untoward aftermath.

What inspired: Trial Vaginal Route but in a wrong case.

LESSONS

- Frozen HP and readiness to switch over to laparotomy
- Taking her as "TRIAL vaginal route" was less disturbing.

CASE 37: VH WITH BSO AND RIGHT BROAD LIGAMENT MYOMECTOMY FOR RIGHT BROAD LIGAMENT FIBROID (BLF)

Name: Mrs. X
Age: 54 years
Parity: 4 FTND
LD: 24 years back.
C/O: Heavy, painful menses with pain in right lower abdomen.
LMP: 10 days back.
Clinically uterus 12 weeks size, mobile and nodular, normal cervix with physiological descent to attempt VH. Right adnexal, firm mass.
Sonography: It revealed uterus with volume of 240 cm^3 with right broad ligament fibroid (BLF) 8 cm × 3.5 cm. Ovaries normal.
Diagnosis: Uterine fibroids with right broad ligament fibroid.
Operation: VH, BSO and broad ligament myomectomy[21] without laparoscopy.
What deters/dissuades: BLF.
Access to vesicouterine peritoneum as well access to the posterior pouch or peritoneal cavity was easy. As per routine, hysterectomy was performed and uterus was freed by cutting all the lateral connections on one side. Traction on free uterus on one side facilitated salpingo-oophorectomy on other side. On naked eye examination, cut open uterus was normal except for its size. This was followed by salpingo-oophorectomy of contralateral normal side and thus complete the hysterectomy with BSO.[7,8] This brought the BLF on the right closer or proximal for the operator. Right BLF was easily felt and seen bulging. Anatomy was respected and the capsule of the fibroid was very carefully cut to enucleate the fibroid (Figs. 1 and 2). Small bleeders were cauterized to ensure hemostasis. Access and enucleation of BLF were straightforward.[3,18,21-22] Hemostasis was checked and vaginal closure done. Blood transfusion was not needed. Hospital stay was 2 days with speedy postoperative recovery.

Histopathology: It showed uterus weighed 260 g, with fibroids. Both ovaries and tubes were normal. Right BLF weighed 80 g. No malignancy.

What inspired: Experience of salpingo-oophorectomy at VH.

LESSONS

1. Concomitant broad ligament myomectomy at VH was easy, easier than salpingo-oophorectomy for endometriotic cyst. The patient was spared an abdominal and/or laparoscopic procedure.[23]
2. Broad ligament myomectomy added flavor.

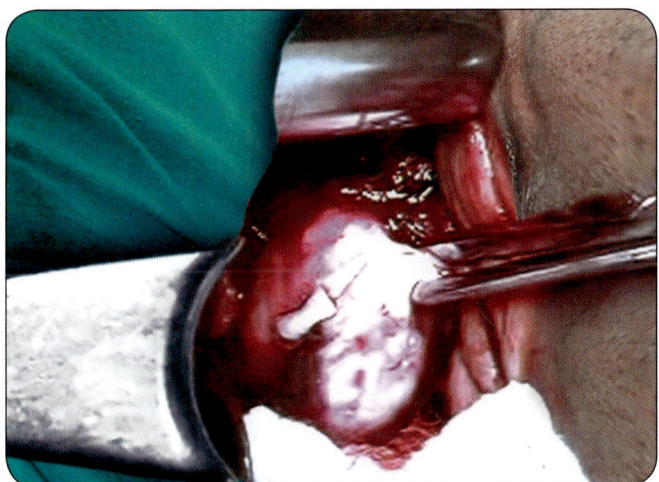

Fig. 1: After an incision of the capsule, the broad ligament fibroid occupying vaginal space is held with Allis' forceps.[21]

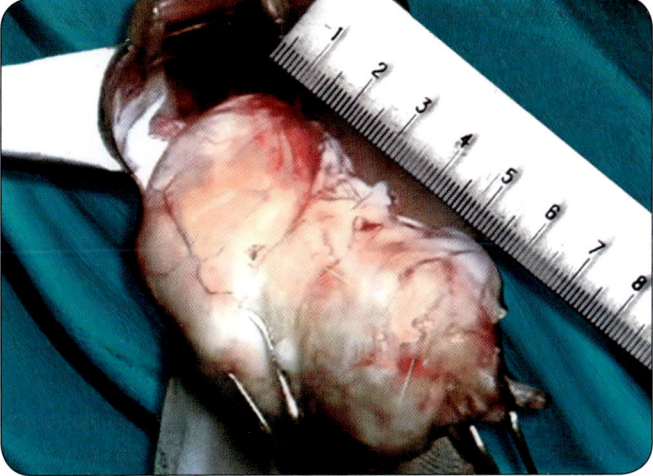

Fig. 2: A broad ligament fibroid of 8 cm size about to be taken out from the operative field.[21]

DISCUSSION FOR BROAD LIGAMENT FIBROID

A BLF is a primary one, lateral to the uterus and it is not an integral part of the uterus.

It is usually well located within the pelvis, lateral to the lateral uterine border and medial to the pelvic wall. Reliable sonography will show ovaries separate from the BLF.

Once the VH is completed or close to completion, adequate space is available for the excision and removal of the BLF. Anxiety and reluctance in approaching a BLF vaginally is unnecessary as the anatomic access is simple and feasible and back up experience of salpingo-oophorectomy at VH will be of great help.

The bulge of a myoma is easier to palpate from medial to lateral, and because of the limitation of the pelvic wall laterally, palpation is easier when a BLF is large. In other words, larger sized BLF is proximal and easier to access from medially. The medial surface of the BLF lies invariably at a lesser distance than the distance at which the ovary lies from the uterus. Surgically, if the operator can reach laterally and distally located IPL vaginally during a salpingo-oophorectomy, it is logical to anticipate access to proximally or medially placed medial surface of the BLF and undertake its extirpation.

The prerequisites for performing concomitant removal of a BLF at VH:
1. Experience of VH and concomitant salpingo-oophorectomy at VH.
2. Fully informed consent.
3. Experienced assistance, a long retractor and fiberoptic light to gain access to the BLF.
4. Attempt as *'Trial vaginal route'*.

Ureter: Even if, anatomically, the ureter is not expected there, it is always worth looking for and ensuring that it is not there before incising the capsule of the BLF.

CASE 38: VH WITH BSO FOR TWISTED LEFT OVARIAN CYST

Name: Mrs. X
Age: 59 years
Parity: 1 FTFD
LD: 23 years back
C/O: Postmenopausal bleeding
LMP: 13 years back

Severe lower abdomen pain with vomiting.

Not obese with no H/O hypertension or diabetes. Tachycardia, lower abdominal tenderness, guarding and mild distension present. Clinically uterus 6 weeks size with restricted mobility. Normal cervix showed physiological descent to attempt vaginal hysterectomy. Left and posterior fornices filled with tender, firm to cystic mass.

Sonography: It showed uterine volume of 100 cm^3 with left ovarian cyst in POD 7.2 cm × 6.3 cm × 7.6 cm, hemorrhagic with clots, without septa and solid area and few twists, reported as left twisted ovarian cyst by a reliable sonologist, Dr Darshana Kshirsagar, Consultant Radiologist, NM Medical Centre, Mumbai, India. Right tube and ovary were normal. Preoperative diagnosis was twisted left ovarian cyst with acute abdomen. Preoperative work out was normal.

Treatment advised was hysterectomy with BSO. Twisted ovarian cyst per se demands laparoscopic surgery or laparotomy and vaginal route is not ever considered for its management.

However on assessing her for VH, clinically cervix and uterus were favorable for hysterectomy. Moot question then was of dealing with "twisted ovarian cyst". Past experience of salpingo-oophorectomy for adnexal pathology including some not so easy, encouraged and inspired to undertake vaginal route.

Diagnosis: Left twisted ovarian cyst.
Operation: VH with BSO. "Trial Vaginal Route".
What deters/dissuades vaginal route: Twisted ovarian cyst and emergency.

Clinically and EUA favored VH. Taken as "Trial Vaginal Route" case.[2,3] VH was straightforward. After uterines were secured as the cyst was on the left side all lateral connections including cornual or upper pedicle were excised on the right side to free the uterus on the right side. Thus the freed uterus from its connections on the right was turned to the left so that the posterior uterine surface faced the operator. This gave ample-free space to visualize the contents in POD and make ovary and tube free from flimsy adhesions. After safe isolation of the operative field alround and covering the area with an isolation sheet, the contents of cyst were aspirated with 16 No needle to debulk the cyst and get it exteriorized. Needle was connected to a suction apparatus. 150 cc of hemorrhagic fluid was easily aspirated. Gravity from head high position, suprapubic pressure and gentle traction on the free uterus to the left showed gangrenous, hemorrhagic, thin-walled cyst on the left with three twists at IPL. Left round ligament was cut as distally or laterally as possible to get an access to IPL and clamp it for salpingo-oophorectomy, which included twisted gangrenous cystic mass[24] (Fig. 1). This was easily possible. It was then followed by prophylactic salpingo-oophorectomy of contralateral normal right tube and ovary, so as to have BSO. This had earlier been consented to by the patient. Cut open uterus showed normal endometrial lining. Blood transfusion was not needed. Hospital stay was 2 days followed by an uneventful speedy recovery.

Histopathology: It showed typical of twisted cyst, totally infracted and gangrenous, reddish brown, hemorrhagic collapsed benign para tubal cyst along with left tube and left ovary. Uterus, right tube and ovary were normal. No malignancy.

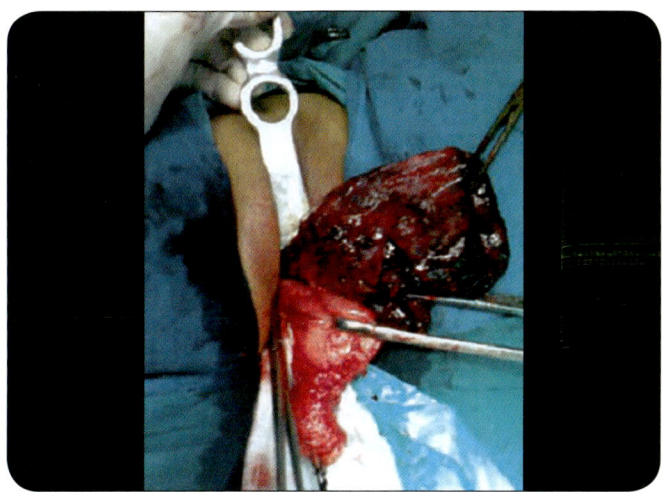

Fig. 1: Twisted ovarian cyst. Uterus with severed nonpathological left lateral connections and intact right upper pedicle showing a debulked, gangrenous and necrotic ovarian cyst measuring 10.5 cm, 8.5 cm and 8.6 cm.
Source: Adapted from reference 24.

What inspired: Major parameters were normal for possible VH.

Back up experience of salpingo-oophorectomy for adnexal pathology at VH.

Crux: Zeal and enthusiasm for rare attempt.

LESSON

- Inspiring to recommend to experienced colleagues, when an opportunity arises.

REFERENCES

1. Sheth SS. The nulliparous patient. In: Sheth SS (Ed). Vaginal Hysterectomy, 2nd edition. New Delhi, India: Jaypee Brothers Medical Publishers (P) Ltd; 2014. pp. 63-71.
2. Sheth SS. Vaginal hysterectomy. In: Studd J (Ed). Progress in Obstetrics and Gynecology, 10th edition. London, UK: Churchill Livingstone; 1993. pp. 317-40.
3. Sheth SS, Paghdiwalla KP, Hajari AR. Vaginal route: a gynaecological route for much more than hysterectomy. Best Pract Res Clin Obstet Gynaecol. 2011;25(2):115-32.
4. Sheth SS. Adnexal pathology at vaginal hysterectomy. In: Sheth SS (Ed). Vaginal Hysterectomy, 2nd edition. New Delhi, India: Jaypee Brothers Medical Publishers (P) Ltd; 2014. pp. 150-62.
5. Sheth SS. Adnexectomy for benign pathology at vaginal hysterectomy without laparoscopic assistance. Br J Obstet Gynecol. 2002;109:1401-5.
6. Sheth SS, Malpani AN. Vaginal hysterectomy following previous caesarean section. Int J Gynecol Obstet. 1995;50:165-9.
7. Sheth SS. The place of oophorectomy at vaginal hysterectomy. Br J Obstet Gynecol. 1991;98:662-6.
8. Sheth SS. The place of oophorectomy at vaginal hysterectomy. Obstet Gynecol Surv. 1992;47:332-3.
9. Kwon JS, Tinker A, Pansegrau G, et al. Prophylactic salpingectomy and delayed oophorectomy as an alternative for BRCA mutation carriers. Obstet Gynecol. 2013;121:14-24.
10. Sheth SS. Vaginal hysterectomy as primary route for morbidly obese women. Acta Obstet Gynecol. 2010;89:971-4.
11. Sheth SS. Management of ovarian dermoid without laparoscopy or laparotomy. Eur J Obstet Gynecol Reprod Biol. 2001;99:106-8.
12. Pardi G, Carminati R, Ferrari MM, et al. Laparoscopically assisted vaginal removal of ovarian dermoid cysts. Obstet Gynecol. 1995;85:129-32.
13. Chapron C, Dubuisson JB. Laparoscopic treatment of ovarian dermoid cyst. Am J obstet Gynecol. 1996;175:234-5.
14. Yoong W, Pillai R. Posterior colpotomy--a retrieval route for solid ovarian tumours. BJOG. 2009;116:465-6.
15. Teng FY, Muzsnai D, Perez R, et al. A comparative study of laparoscopy and colpotomy for the removal of ovarian dermoid cysts. Obstet Gynecol. 1996;87:1009-13.
16. Sheth SS. Vaginal dimple--a sign of ovarian endometriosis. J Obstet Gynecol. 1991;11;292.
17. Sheth SS. A surgical window to access the obliterated posterior cul-de-sac at vaginal hysterectomy. Int J Gynecol Obstet. 2009;107:244-7.
18. Sheth SS. Newer perspectives. In: Sheth SS (Ed). Vaginal Hysterectomy, 2nd edition. New Delhi, India: Jaypee Brothers Medical Publishers (P) Ltd; 2014. pp. 225-34.
19. Zanagnolo V, Magrina JF. Vaginal hysterectomy for carcinoma of the endometrium. In: Sheth SS (Ed). Vaginal Hysterectomy, 2nd edition. New Delhi, India: Jaypee Brothers Medical Publishers (P) Ltd; 2014. pp. 216-24.
20. Gultekin E, Gultekin OE, Cingillioglu B, et al. The value of frozen section evaluation in the management of borderline ovarian tumors. J Cancer Res Ther. 2011;7:416-20.
21. Sheth SS. Broad ligament myomectomy at vaginal hysterectomy without laparoscopic assistance. J Gynecol Surg. 2007;23:133-41.
22. Macleod D, Howkins J (Eds). Hysterectomy for cervical and broad-ligament myoma. In: Bonney's Gynaecological Surgery, 7th edition. London, UK: William Clowes and Sons Ltd; 1964. pp. 253-76.
23. Sheth SS. Observations from a FIGO Past President on vaginal hysterectomy and related surgery by the vaginal route. Int J Gynecol Obstet. 2016;135:1-4.
24. Sheth SS, Srinivasan R, Darda P. Twisted ovarian cyst treated via the vaginal route. Int J Gynecol Obstet. 2011;113:245-6.

Section 4: NULLIPARA AND VAGINAL HYSTERECTOMY

"Being ignorant is not so much a shame, as being unwilling to learn."
—Benjamin Franklin

CASES

Dr Shirish S Sheth

Case 39: *VH in Nullipara with Intact Hymen*
Case 40: *VH with Uterine Debulking*
Case 41: *VH with Uterine Debulking Plus Right Ovarian Endometrial Cystectomy (H/O Myomectomy)*
Case 42: *VH with BSO for Bilateral Large Hydrosalpinx*
Case 43: *VH Plus Vaginal Cuff with BSO in Obese, Diabetic with Endometrial Cancer*
Case 44: *VH with BSO for Twisted Left Ovarian Cyst*

CASE 39: VH IN NULLIPARA WITH INTACT HYMEN

Name: Miss X
Age: 22 years
Parity: Nullipara

The parents complained that it was impossible to take care of menstruation and maintain menstrual hygiene of their mentally compromised 22-year-old daughter. The menstrual cycles were regular and normal. They were keen to have her uterus removed if possible.[1-4]

She was mentally compromised with IQ (intelligence quotient) of 24 and mental age corresponding to 3 years. Systemic findings were normal though it was not easy to examine her. Clinically, the pelvic examination was not done. Pelvic findings were expected to be normal as abdominopelvic sonography findings were normal. Uterine volume was 35 cm³. The desire to perform hysterectomy vaginally is important, as the uterine size and other pelvic findings were normal, favoring a vaginal route for hysterectomy.

Diagnosis: Mentally compromised patient.
Operation: Vaginal hysterectomy (VH).
Facts which deter/dissuade VH: Nulliparity with intact hymen (Fig. 1).

First pelvic examination that she had was under anesthesia. A small speculum was inserted and rotated through 360° twice or thrice to break the intact hymen, to increase the introital dimension and facilitate vaginal laxity. This was followed by pelvic examination under anesthesia (EUA) to confirm normalcy and absence of any contraindication to VH. This was the first pelvic examination the patient ever had. There was less space for hysterectomy but sufficient enough to start. Thereafter, hysterectomy was carefully and gradually proceeded with. One needs to exercise both extra care and gentleness with the use of a small Sim's speculum instead of the bigger self-retaining large Auward's speculum, small vaginal wall retractors and bladder retractor, an experienced assistant, and the appropriate technique for securing the pedicles. The author secures pedicles with sutures by the clampless technique, which makes it easier because space is at a premium and it is a technique that he regularly practices (Figs. 2A and B).[5-6] Thus, without difficulty the hysterectomy was completed. The tubes and ovaries were normal. As expected, naked eye examination of the cut uterus was normal.

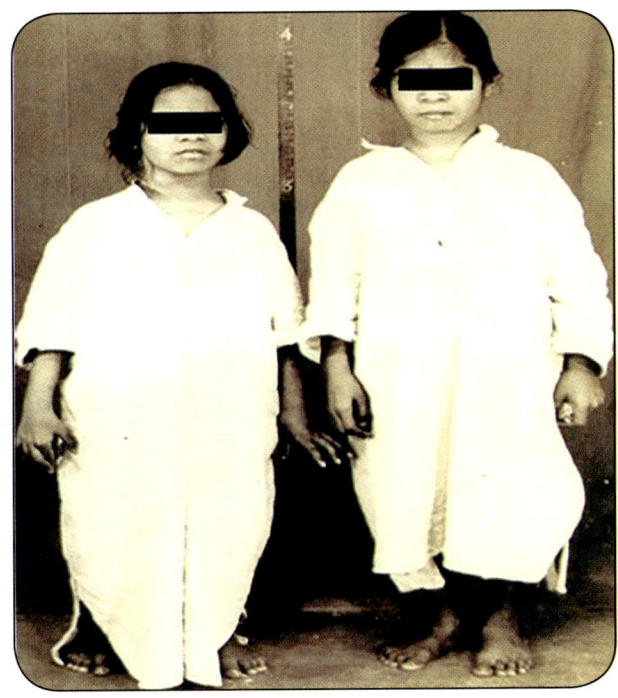

Fig. 1: Two young women with mental age of 2 years and 4 years, respectively, with intact hymen.[7]

Hemostasis was checked and vaginal closure done. Blood loss was less than 50 cc. Blood transfusion was not needed. Postoperatively, the patient was put in a special bed to restrict her movements. The same evening, liquids were started orally and she was made to walk. As the abdomen was intact, the parents were very happy and very cooperative, without any anxiety of wound care. The hospital stay was 3 days as desired by her parents. She made an uneventful, speedy recovery.

Histopathology (HP): Uterus weighed 35 g. Endometrium secretory. No pathology found.

The author has by now performed more than 125 vaginal hysterectomies without a single failure for mentally compromised or disabled patients with intact hymen except in two. When more space is needed, there should be no hesitation in giving a mini-episiotomy or small Schuchardt's incision to enlarge the available space. This was done by the author in the initial period, in 8 out of the first 20 cases and thereafter never needed.[5,7]

What inspired: Past experience.

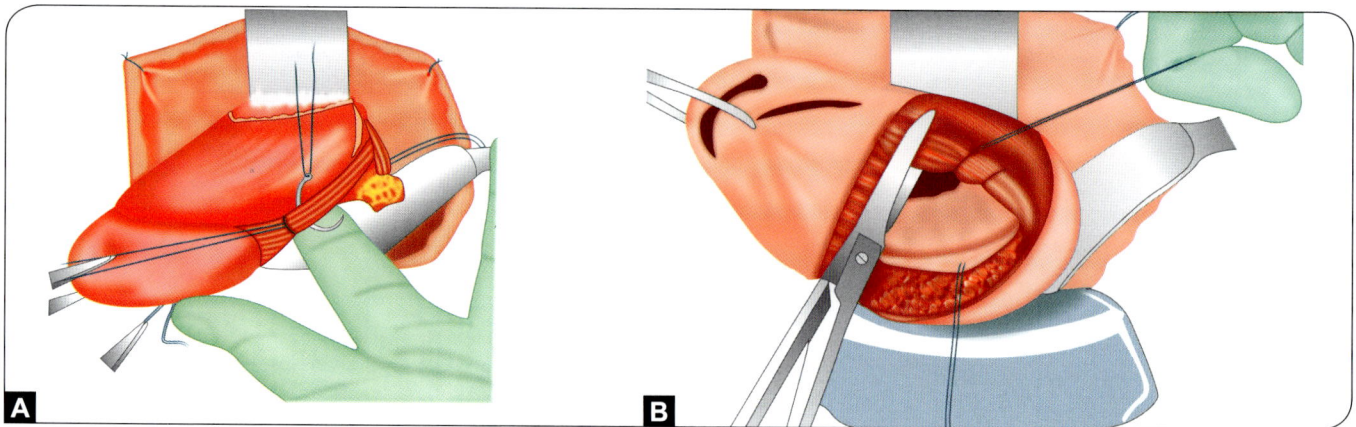

Figs. 2A and B: Suture technique (clampless method): Needle with the suturing material that goes around the tissue to secure, shows finger hooking around uterosacral ligament.[6]

LESSONS

- Intact hymen and therefore nulliparity should never dissuade VH.
- It gives immense experience and serves as a morale booster to remove "nulliparity" as a deterring factor from the mind.

The author demonstrated the above surgery on a similar patient at a VH workshop at Shimoga, Karnataka, India which was very well received.

The parents, mother in particular, was very troubled and overstrained during the daughter's menstrual cycles. The mother moved like her shadow to ensure that her daughter was not physically attacked and harassed by outsiders. To spare her from unwanted pregnancy, laparoscopic tubal sterilization[1] can be done but that does not solve the main problem of menstrual hygiene. The topic of sterilization of such mentally retarded or disabled women is also controversial. Experience in some countries favors hysterectomy[4] as it will eradicate the major problem, i.e. menstrual hygiene care and improve the quality of life. In psychiatry, individual with IQ of 25 or less is called IDIOT and with IQ between 26 and 50 as IMBECILE.

Nullipara and particularly with an intact hymen induce most gynecologists to perform total laparoscopic hysterectomy (TLH) or open the abdomen for hysterectomy. However, for a normal size uterus without pelvic pathology and obstetric trauma in the past, the vaginal route should be an ideal choice. It will spare the abdomen and thus reduce postoperative wound dressing, etc. in a highly disturbed, non co-operative patient.

Zeal and, enthusiasm on the part of the gynecologist and absence of contraindications favors the vaginal route for hysterectomy. To convince parents for a vaginal approach is extremely easy as they want hysterectomy for their child with minimum postoperative care and anxiety, shorter hospital stay, rapid recovery without an external cut and minimal wound care and they get those advantages.[8,9] With numerous mentally challenged women, the least invasive VH can become a boon for India and China and to gynecologists interested in the vaginal route for hysterectomy to master. It will also provide a great boost to deal with VH in nullipara in the future.

CASE 40: VH WITH UTERINE DEBULKING

Name: Mrs. X
Age: 46 years
Parity: Nullipara.

Not obese with no history of (H/O) hypertension or diabetes.

Uterus 18–20 weeks size, nodular with large fibroid. Cervix was favorable for attempting VH. Fornices were clear.

Sonography: It gave uterine volume of 688 cm^3 with 14 cm × 10.7 cm × 8.5 cm uterine dimensions,[10] multiple fibroids with a large posterior wall fibroid. Tubes and ovaries were normal. Taken as "Trial VH" case.[11]

Diagnosis: Uterine fibroids.
Operation: VH.
What deters or dissuades VH: Large uterus in a nullipara.

Vaginal hysterectomy started as usual, after uterines were secured and cervix well bisected followed by morcellation-n-enucleation of small and large fibroids and morcellation of uterine adenomyotic walls without difficulty.[7,9,10,12-15] Thus, hysterectomy was completed. Normal tubes and ovaries were preserved.

Hemostasis was checked and vaginal closure was done. Blood transfusion was not needed. Hospital stay was 2 days with an uneventful speedy recovery.

Histopathology: It showed uterus weighed 840 g with multiple fibroids and severe adenomyosis.

What inspired:
- Physiological cervical descent plus experience of debulking.

LESSONS

- Nulliparity with large uterus
- Success leads to progress.

CASE 41: VH WITH UTERINE DEBULKING PLUS RIGHT OVARIAN ENDOMETRIAL CYSTECTOMY (H/O MYOMECTOMY)

Name: Mrs. X
Age: 38 years
Parity: Nullipara
H/O: Abdominal myomectomies
Complains of (C/O): Heavy and painful menses with lower abdominal pain.

Clinically freely mobile uterus of 16 weeks size without nodularity. Healthy cervix with favorable descent to attempt VH. Fornices were clear except right with a soft to firm mass. ?Endometriotic ovarian cyst.

Sonography: It showed uterus with 8.4 cm × 9.8 cm × 9.2 cm uterine dimensions, volume 409 cm^3. Right ovarian cyst 4 cm × 3 cm, endometriotic. Rest of the abdominopelvic findings were normal. CA125 was 266.

Diagnosis: Severe adenomyosis with right ovarian endometrial cyst.

Operation: VH with bilateral salpingectomy and right ovarian cystectomy.

What deters or dissuades VH: Nulliparity plus endometriotic cyst.

After uterines were secured, the cervix was bisected and adenomyotic uterus was debulked. Chocolaty material exuded also from the serosal surface of the uterine walls. Debulking of adenomyotic uterine walls was totally by morcellation with nothing to enucleate.[12,14] Surely, morcellating is tougher than enucleating a fibroid. Small intestines and omentum were adherent to the uterine fundus because of myomectomies in the past. Adhesions were carefully separated to free the uterus, tube and ovary all-round.[15-17] Uterus was distinctly adenomyotic without fibroids.

Right ovary with the small endometriotic cyst was excised and remaining healthy ovary was preserved.

Both tubes were hematosalpinx (missed on sonography), which needed bilateral salpingectomy. Thus, vaginal hysterectomy, right ovarian cystectomy and bilateral salpingectomy was done.[17-19] Left normal ovary was also preserved. She was keen to preserve the ovaries, if healthy. After checking hemostasis, vaginal closure was done. Hospital stay was 3 days. Postoperatively she had uneventful speedy recovery with normal CA125 after 4 weeks.[20]

Histopathology: It showed uterus weighed 470 g with severe adenomyosis and endometriotic cyst of right ovary. Left tube was endometriotic and right tube without pathology. No malignancy.

What inspired: Experience of hysterectomies in nullipara and concomitant salpingo-oophorectomy at VH.

LESSONS

- Large uterus, nullipara and endometriotic cyst dealt with.
- Raised CA125 mainly due to severe adenomyosis and partly due to ovarian endometriotic cyst.

CASE 42: VH WITH BSO FOR BILATERAL LARGE HYDROSALPINX

Name: Mrs. X
Age: 58 years
Parity: Nullipara
C/O: Postmenopausal spotting for 2 months and pain in lower abdomen.
Last menstrual period (LMP): 8 years back
Mildly obese (BMI 31) with no H/O hypertension or diabetes. She had a normal size uterus with restricted mobility and a normal cervix which had physiological descent to favor VH. Cystic swellings in both lateral fornices, tender and free.
Sonography: Revealed a normal size uterus with volume 38 cm^3, endometrial thickness of 3 mm plus bilateral hydrosalpinx (right 4.6 cm × 3 cm and left 8 cm × 3 cm). Both ovaries normal.
Diagnosis: Bilateral hydrosalpinx.
Operation: VH with bilateral salpingo-oophorectomy (BSO).
What deters/dissuades VH: Nulliparity.
Examination under anesthesia: It confirmed that she was fit for a 'Trial vaginal route' case as VH appeared possible.[10,19] After the uterines were secured, normal size uterus was easily fully bisected into two halves, each with intact upper pedicle including the hydrosalpinx on both sides.

Both tubes and ovaries were mildly adherent to each other but free from surrounding area. This was lysed to free both the tubes and ovaries.

Head high and gravity with suprapubic pressure helped to deliver and exteriorize the hydrosalpinx. The surgical field was well isolated with a sterile plastic sheet. The large left hydrosalpinx was reduced in size by aspiration. Traction on the left half of the uterus gave easy access to the infundibulopelvic ligament (IPL) to perform left salpingo-oophorectomy. This provided ample-free space to complete contralateral salpingo-oophorectomy with traction on the remaining right half of the uterus in a similar fashion and thus complete the hysterectomy with BSO.[16-19] Cut open uterus showed normal endometrium. Both salpingo-oophorectomies included the tubes with hydrosalpinx. In both, the round ligaments were cut as laterally as possible to facilitate traction on the bisected half uterus. Blood transfusion was not needed. Hospital stay was 2 days followed by an uneventful, speedy recovery.

Histopathology: It showed bilateral hydrosalpinx (4+ cm and 8+ cm size) without malignancy. The uterus, cervix and both ovaries were normal. The uterus weighed 46 g. No malignancy.

What inspired: Experience of concomitant salpingo-oophorectomy at VH and hysterectomies in nullipara.

LESSONS

1. Nulliparity should never dissuade VH.
2. Close to completion of hysterectomy, ample free space becomes available to deal with adnexal pathology.

CASE 43: VH PLUS VAGINAL CUFF WITH BSO IN OBESE, DIABETIC WITH ENDOMETRIAL CANCER

Name: Mrs. X
Age: 54 years
Parity: Nullipara
LMP: 2 years back
C/O: Recurrent postmenopausal bleeding.

The patient was obese [body mass index (BMI) 35] with H/O diabetes but not hypertension. Clinically uterus 6 weeks size, healthy cervix with physiological descent to attempt VH and fornices were clear. She needed "superflexion" position for careful speculum examination to reduce the effects of morbid obesity[21] (Fig. 1).

Sonography findings: It showed uterine volume of 110 cm³, endometrial thickness 10 mm and normal pelvic findings.

She was referred after H/O hysteroscopy plus dilatation and curettage (D&C) and diagnosis of well-differentiated endometrioid adenocarcinoma for further treatment.

Invariably, advice would have been to have abdominal access, laparotomy or laparoscopic surgery. Hoping for less myometrial invasion, accentuated by the presence of diabetes and obesity favored an attempt to do VH.[6,19,22] Management was discussed at length, pros and cons explained including sparing of opening the abdomen or need to open it, if frozen HP study of the uterus indicated.

Diagnosis: Well-differentiated endometrial carcinoma.
Operation: VH with vaginal cuff plus BSO.
What deters/dissuades: If myometrial invasion is half or more.

Vaginal hysterectomy with vaginal cuff of 3 cm and hysterectomy with unilateral salpingo-oophorectomy was performed and sent for frozen HP study. Fluid from pouch of Douglas was taken for cytology study. Further management depended on frozen HP report of myometrial invasion by malignancy in the hysterectomized uterus. Meanwhile, contralateral salpingo-oophorectomy was completed (Age: 54 years.). Frozen HP study reported 2 mm invasion out of 15 mm myometrial wall/thickness,

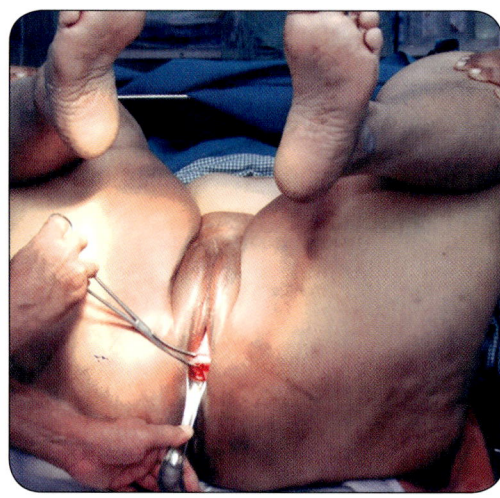

Fig. 1: Superflexion position. The patient's hands keep both feet apart and thus provide a clear view of the vulva and vaginal area.[21]

much less than 50%. This ruled out lymph node removal and therefore, laparotomy or laparoscopic surgery and spared her from the greater invasion of opening the abdomen or 4–5 punctures and resultant greater morbidity in an obese, diabetic woman.[8,23-27] After checking hemostasis, vaginal closure done.

Blood transfusion was not needed. Hospital stay was 2 days with an uneventful postoperative speedy recovery. Later, the radiotherapist opined that she did not need any postoperative radiotherapy.

Histopathology: It showed uterus of 136 g, showed small unhealthy endometrial area, otherwise normal. Myometrial invasion of barely 3 mm out of 15 mm uterine wall. Tubes, ovaries and vaginal cuff were normal.

What inspired: High risk for abdominal surgery.

LESSON

- Trial vaginal route and frozen HP report were immensely useful.

CASE 44: VH WITH BSO FOR TWISTED LEFT OVARIAN CYST

Please See on page 73 Under Section 3: Vaginal Hysterectomy with Adnexal Pathology, Case 38.

REFERENCES

1. Van Der Merwe JV, Roux JP. Sterilisation of mentally retarded person. Obstet Gynecol Surv. 1987;42:489-93.
2. Passer A, Rauh J, Chamberlain A, et al. Issues in fertility control for mentally retarded female adolescents: II. Parental attitudes toward sterilization. Pediatrics. 1984;73(4):451-4.
3. Kaunitz AM, Thompson RJ, Kaunitz KK. Mental retardation: a controversial indication for hysterectomy. Obstet Gynecol. 1986;68(3):436-8.
4. Wheeless CR. Abdominal hysterectomy for surgical sterilization in the mentally retarded: a review of parental opinion. Am J Obstet Gynecol. 1975;122(7):872-5.
5. Sheth SS, Malpani AN. Vaginal hysterectomy for the management of menstruation in mentally retarded women. Int J Gynecol Obstet. 1991;35:319-21.
6. Sheth SS. Vaginal hysterectomy. Best Pract Res Clin Obstet Gynaecol. 2005;19(3):307-32.
7. Sheth SS. The nulliparous patient. In: Sheth SS (Ed). Vaginal Hysterectomy, 2nd edition. New Delhi, India: Jaypee Brothers Medical Publishers (P) Ltd; 2014. pp. 63-71.
8. Nieboer TE, Johnson N, Lethaby A, et al. Surgical approach to hysterectomy for benign gynecological disease. Cochrane Database Syst Rev. 2009;(3):CD003677.
9. Agostini A, Bretelle F, Cravello L, et al. Vaginal hysterectomy in nulliparous women without prolapse: a prospective comparative study. BJOG. 2003;110:515-8.
10. Sheth SS, Shah NM. Preoperative sonographic estimation of uterine volume: an aid to determine the route of hysterectomy. J Gynecol Surg. 2002;18:13-22.
11. Sheth SS. Vaginal hysterectomy. In: Studd J (Ed). Progress in Obstetrics and Gynaecology, 10th edition. London, UK: Churchill Livingstone; 1993. pp. 317-40.
12. Tohic AL, Dhainaut C, Yazbeck C, et al. Hysterectomy for benign uterine pathology among women without previous vaginal delivery. Obstet Gynecol. 2008;111:829-37.
13. Kovac RS. Intramyometrial coring as an adjunct to vaginal hysterectomy. Obstet Gynecol. 1986;67:131-6.
14. Sheth SS. Rathi MR. Uterine fibroids. In: Sheth SS (Ed). Vaginal Hysterectomy, 2nd edition. New Delhi, India: Jaypee Brothers Medical Publishers (P) Ltd; 2014. pp. 72-89.
15. Benedetti-Panici P, Maneschi F, Cutillo G, et al. Surgery by minilaparotomy in benign gynecologic disease. Obstet Gynecol. 1996;87(3):456-9.
16. Sheth SS. Concomitant salpingo-oophorectomy at vaginal hysterectomy. In: Sheth SS (Ed). Vaginal Hysterectomy, 2nd edition. New Delhi, India: Jaypee Brothers Medical Publishers (P) Ltd; 2014. pp. 137-49.
17. Sheth SS. Adnexectomy for benign pathology at vaginal hysterectomy without laparoscopic assistance. Br. J Obstet Gynecol. 2002;109:1401-5.
18. Sheth SS. Adnexal pathology at vaginal hysterectomy. In: Sheth SS (Ed). Vaginal Hysterectomy, 2nd edition. New Delhi, India: Jaypee Brothers Medical Publishers (P) Ltd; 2014. pp. 150-62.
19. Sheth SS, Paghdiwalla KP, Hajari AR. Vaginal route: a gynaecological route for much more than hysterectomy. Best Pract Res Clin Obstet Gynaecol. 2011;25(2):115-32.
20. Sheth SS, Ray SS. Severe adenomyosis and CA125. J Obstet Gynecol. 2014;34:79-81.
21. Sheth SS. Superflexion position for difficult speculum examination. Int J Gynaecol Obstet. 2013;121:92-3.
22. Sheth SS. Vaginal hysterectomy as primary route for morbidly obese women. Acta Obstet Gynecol. 2010;89:971-4.
23. Massi G, SaVino L, Susni T, et al. Vaginal hysterectomy vs abdominal hysterectomy for the treatment or stage 1 endometrial adenocarcinoma. Am J Obstet Gynecol. 1996;174:1320-26.
24. ASTEC Study group Efficacy of systematic pelvic lymphadenectomy in endometrial cancer (MRC ASTEC trial): a randomized study. Lancet. 2009;373:125-36.
25. Jones HW. New developments in the surgical management of early endometrial cancer. Obstet Gynecol. 2009;114:2-3.
26. Zanagnolo V, Magrina JF. Carcinoma of the endometrium treated only by vaginal route. Best Pract Res Clin Obstet Gynaecol. 2011;25:239-45.
27. Zanagnolo V, Magrina JF. Vaginal hysterectomy for carcinoma of the endometrium. In: Sheth SS (Ed). Vaginal Hysterectomy, 2nd edition. New Delhi, India: Jaypee Brothers Medical Publishers (P) Ltd; 2014. pp. 216-24.

Section 5
VAGINAL HYSTERECTOMY FOR ENDOMETRIAL CANCER

"Better put a strong fence round the top of the cliff than an ambulance down in the valley."
—Richard Nichols

CASES

Dr Shirish S Sheth

Introduction
Case 45: VH Plus Vaginal Cuff with BSO: Postmenopausal Bleeder with Endometrial Complex Hyperplasia with Atypia
Case 46: VH Plus Vaginal Cuff with BSO: Postmenopausal Bleeder with Corpus Cancer Syndrome for Endometrial Cancer (CA)
Case 47: VH Plus Vaginal Cuff with BSO for Endometrial CA
Case 48: VH Plus Vaginal Cuff with BSO: Postmenopausal Bleeder with Corpus Cancer Syndrome. Failed "Trial Vaginal Route". Abdominal Surgery for LNR for Endometrial CA
Case 49: VH Plus Vaginal Cuff with BSO for Endometrial Complex Hyperplasia with Atypia. Corpus CA Syndrome Plus a History of Cardiac Bypass
Case 50: VH Plus Vaginal Cuff with BSO for Well-differentiated Endometrial Adenocarcinoma
Case 51: VH Plus Vaginal Cuff with BSO: Postmenopausal Bleeder with Endometrial CA with History of Two Caesarean Sections Followed by Incisional Hernia Repair
Case 52: VH Plus Vaginal Cuff with BSO Plus Laparoscopic Cholecystectomy for Postmenopausal Bleeder with Multiple Gallstones
Case 53: Laparoscopic Cholecystectomy and VH Plus Vaginal Cuff with BSO: "Failed Trial Vaginal Route Case" Abdominal LNR for Endometrial CA

INTRODUCTION

Postmenopausal Bleeding and Endometrial Histopathology

- Postmenopausal vaginal bleeding with abnormal endometrial thickness (ET) → Vaginal hysterectomy (VH) with or without bilateral salpingo-oophorectomy (BSO) → Frozen histopathology (HP) → Simple or complex hyperplasia with OR without atypia. No malignancy.
- Postmenopausal bleeding with abnormal ET → VH with or without BSO → Frozen HP → Polyp. No malignancy.
- Postmenopausal bleeding with abnormal ET → VH with or without BSO → Frozen HP → Cancer (CA) → Myometrial invasion (MI) less than half OR less than 50%.
- Postmenopausal bleeding with abnormal ET → VH with or without BSO → Frozen HP → "CA" → MI half OR more.
- Postmenopausal bleeding with abnormal ET HP → Hysteroscopy plus dilation and curettage (D & C) → Endometrial "CA" → VH with BSO. Lymph node removal (LNR) only if MI is half or more, OR if required.
- Perimenopausal abnormal uterine bleeding (AUB) in an obese woman with hypertension and/or diabetes with abnormal ET → VH with or without BSO → Frozen HP. Further management will depend on the frozen HP report.

Those postmenopausal bleeders who do not need hysterectomy, but are with abnormal ET should be subjected to hysteroscopy plus D&C and endometrial HP to decide further treatment.

However, those with abnormal ET who need hysterectomy even otherwise, they can straightaway, without hysteroscopy plus curettage undergo VH with cuff of vagina plus BSO, if indicated. They will be spared of hysteroscopy plus D&C or endometrial curettage and will have a hysterectomized uterus for frozen HP study to not only exclude malignancy but if malignant also provide extent of the MI. A significant number of those showing endometrial cancer, adenocarcinoma or endometrioid, well or moderately differentiated, are with MI less than half and therefore do not need LNR and are spared from the further surgery of laparotomy or laparoscopic surgery except BSO in most VH. Needless to say, they need good and careful counseling and well-informed consent besides a reliable histopathologist. Those with MI of half or more (50% or more)[1] or poorly differentiated or serous cell carcinoma or clear cell carcinoma or sarcoma need LNR for which abdomen is accessed.[2-5] All do not require LNR and thus significant numbers of women are spared from more invasive abdominal surgery and all of them from hysteroscopy plus D&C.

Treatment that early endometrial cancer commonly requires is hysterectomy plus vaginal cuff with BSO. Selective cases need additionally lymph nodes removal and more and similarly, select cases may not need salpingo-oophorectomy. For endometrial "CA", should hysterectomy be always via abdominal surgery or can one undertake less vaginal route for select cases? It is very unlikely that oncosurgeons, including most of "Gynec" oncosurgeons, would think of the vaginal route for endometrial "CA". Interestingly, large trials for the management of endometrial CA are that of abdominal versus laparoscopic hysterectomy emphasizing minimally invasive surgery but without even mention of the vaginal route. Is it lack of knowledge or indifference? It is important to note that there is something like a vaginal route—a gynecological route, provided one is interested in the best interests of women.

Massi, Inguilla, Krige, Quinlan and Magrina[5-12] are in favor of VH as and when indicated.

SALPINGO-OOPHORECTOMY AT VAGINAL HYSTERECTOMY

Removal of ovaries or conservation is always discussed at length preoperatively, more so in cases needing frozen HP study of the just removed uterus. Counseling and well-informed consent are essential. BSO is preferred if frozen HP report is uterine malignancy. However, it is not mandatory to remove ovaries in some select cases. In absence of malignancy, conservation or removal will depend on several factors just as in other women of a similar age.

The author prefers to remove the uterus along with one-sided salpingo-oophorectomy after cutting round ligament distally. Which sided? Prefer to have removal of uterus along with pathological adnexa, if so. Thereafter, it is vital to cut the round ligament as laterally as possible to perform contralateral salpingo-oophorectomy.

Whilst the uterus is undergoing frozen HP study, operator completes the contralateral salpingo-oophorectomy of normal adnexal side and thus BSO—one along with uterus earlier and other thereafter. Contralateral salpingo-oophorectomy makes good use of the available time while careful frozen HP study report is awaited.

LYMPH NODE REMOVAL

Even if malignancy does exist, significant numbers of cases of "CA" endometrium do not require LNR and therefore abdominal access.[13-18]

A trial of more than 1,400 women in the United Kingdom (UK), showed no difference in survival with LNR for apparent uterine-confined disease. An Italian trial of 514 reported the same as that of UK's trial. LNR in women with early endometrial CA will not improve either survival or recurrence rate.[2,3] Study of 151,089 women at 1,336 hospitals. 65% LNR, 34% no LNR. LNR is associated with a modest, if any, effect on survival for women with endometrial CA.[6]

Often abdominal route is chosen, because:
- If it is a cancer case. Even today 60–70% hysterectomies done for benign uterine conditions are abdominal and not vaginal or laparoscopic—something scientifically undesirable and fallacious
- To some, cancer means LNR and therefore
- Cancer means salpingo-oophorectomy is "MUST" and therefore
- Cancer cases mostly go to oncosurgeons, and for oncosurgeons, vaginal route almost does not exist. Actually most "Gynec" oncosurgeons do not perform a straightforward hysterectomy vaginally even for CIN III of cervix when required
- Nonavailability of laparoscope and/or laparoscopic surgeons
- Frozen HP facility may not be available at many centers
- Gynecologist himself or herself though regularly performing VH is unprepared for the LNR, in case frozen HP indicates.

However the picture can change and change drastically, in favor of the patient when a gynecologist experienced with VH with concomitant BSO is also competent to deal abdominally with removal of lymph nodes, if required.

Crux for the operator lies in:
- Experience of vaginal hysterectomies with concomitant BSO
- Reliable frozen HP report (degree of MI, if cancerous)
- Facility to switch over to laparotomy or laparoscopic surgery, if required.

Advantages of vaginal route:
- The least invasive and in the best interests of the patient.
- If frozen HP shows MI of less than half or less than 50%, she does not need LNR and therefore does not need laparotomy or laparoscopy except for poorly differentiated or clear cell cancer or serous cell cancer or sarcoma, etc.
- Undertaking postmenopausal bleeders or recurrent bleeders with abnormal ET, who as such need hysterectomy for one or other indications OR those after hysteroscopy plus D&C showing endometrial complex hyperplasia with atypia or endometrial malignancy. This is a new door for many or a door that has remained unopened.
- Malignancy with MI less than half do not require more than hysterectomy with BSO in most cases.

When abdominal access: Open the abdomen or laparoscopic surgery:
- When LNR is required
- BSO is not possible vaginally
- Vaginal hysterectomy fails
- Complication indicates.

However, the word "cancer" is more than sufficient for opening of the abdomen. Be assured that it is unlikely that an oncosurgeon will take the vaginal route for hysterectomy or consider to go by frozen HP study of the removed uterus and attempt to spare abdomen from either opening with large vertical sub-umbilical incision or several small cuts for laparoscopic surgery. On one side, we are looking for minimally invasive surgery, and on the other side, even when abdomen does not need to be opened, it is opened for abdominal hysterectomy on excuse of malignancy or even for more than 60% benign conditions. For some, their dictionary does not contain word "Pfannenstiel".

LAPAROSCOPIC SURGERY

Laparoscopic surgeons are either indifferent or selectively ignorant to consider that in select women with endometrial CA, full treatment can be given per via naturales with much less invasion.

The important question to gynecologists as well as surgeons is that for his/her mother or sister with history of (H/O) hypertension, diabetes, obesity and/or high risk, will he recommend vaginal surgery for complex endometrial hyperplasia with atypia or well differentiated early endometrial adenocarcinoma or endometrioid CA invading myometrium but much less than half of full thickness?[5,11,13,18]

Cuff Removal

All said and done, removal of cuff is and can be advantageous.[19] Mariani et al.[15] report 3% vaginal cuff recurrence. Controversies exist but Creasman[16] clearly mentions in TeLinde's Operative Book in favor of cuff removal in contrast to Hacker and Friedlander[18] who are not in favor of cuff removal. Poor disease-free survival is associated with high tumor grade and without cuff removal. There is no disadvantage or minus side of cuff removal except bit of additional surgery and a bit of shortening of the vagina. For "CA" one does not and should not consider them.

Preparing cuff is not difficult as posterior part of vaginal cuff is always as such available when pouch of Douglas (POD) is accessed. For anterior vaginal wall, careful higher transverse incision is made to separate the vaginal wall from underlying fascia covering the bladder from distal to proximal of external cervical os or from incision site towards external os of cervix—opposite direction of what is done for anterior colporrhaphy.[13]

WHEN TO DISCHARGE AFTER SURGERY?

Hysterectomy vaginally with BSO done for endometrial "CA" per se does not need or demand extra stay when compared with VH for AUB due to benign pathology, i.e. she can comfortably go home after 24 hours.[20-22] One does not have to prove anything or make "show" by discharging earlier than that. Imposed earlier discharge does not make surgery less invasive but speaks of a woman's reserve and the surgeon's attitude. This will spare her from unnecessary anxiety and telephone calls to nurse and/or doctor. I prefer to discharge the patient after 24–36 hours and also prefer the patient ask for her discharge from the hospital rather than otherwise.

Stay will be longer when abdomen is opened or big cystocele is repaired with VH and patient does not want to go home because of self-retaining (SR) catheter OR similarly, when stress urinary incontinence (SUI) repair is done, prefer not to keep her in the hospital only because of an SR catheter. She can certainly go home with an SR catheter and follow-up can be carefully looked into.

Stovall et al.[20] advocate VH as an outdoor procedure with average hospital stay of 9.4 hours. However, every woman going home early or in less than 24 hours was visited by a social worker/nurse for few days. The author learnt from that publication to telephone every woman undergoing VH after her discharge from the hospital for 1–3 days or more if required. Enquiring was made of her well-being and response to routine queries like pain or spotting or minimal bleeding or having not passed a stool, etc. This gives immense satisfaction to the operated woman, solves her queries and she feels that the doctor is deeply concerned about her. The telephone call may be made by the gynecologist or his experienced staff person. I would strongly recommend this practice as it strengthens the ties between doctor and patient for decades. VH done for "CA" endometrium is not different except for a cuff and mostly BSO.

REFERENCES

1. Pecorelli S. Revised FIGO staging for carcinoma of the vulva, cervix, and endometrium. Int J Gynaecol Obstet. 2009;105(2):103-4.
2. ASTEC study group, Kitchener H, Swart AM, et al. Efficacy of systematic pelvic lymphadenectomy in endometrial cancer (MRC ASTEC trial): a randomised study. Lancet. 2009;373(9658):125-36.
3. Benedetti Panici P, Basile S, Maneschi F, et al. Systematic pelvic lymphadenectomy vs. no lymphadenectomy in early-stage endometrial carcinoma: randomized clinical trial. J Natl Cancer Inst. 2008;100(23):1707-16.
4. Jones HW 3rd. New developments in the surgical management of early endometrial cancer. Obstet Gynecol. 2009;114(1):2-3.
5. Zanagnolo V, Magrina JF. Vaginal hysterectomy for carcinoma of the endometrium. In: Sheth SS (Ed). Vaginal Hysterectomy, 2nd edition. New Delhi, India: Jaypee Brothers Medical Publishers (P) Ltd; 2014. pp. 216-24.
6. Wright JD, Huang Y, Burke WM, et al. Influence of lymphadenectomy on survival for early-stage endometrial cancer. Obstet Gynecol. 2016;127(1):109-18.
7. Massi G, Savino L, Susini T. Vaginal hysterectomy versus abdominal hysterectomy for the treatment of stage I endometrial adenocarcinoma. Am J Obstet Gynecol. 1996;174(4):1320-6.
8. Ingiulla W, Cosmi EV. Vaginal hysterectomy for the treatment of cancer of the corpus uteri. Am J Obstet Gynecol. 1968;100(4):541-3.
9. Krige CF. Vaginal Hysterectomy and Genital Prolapse Repair. A Contribution to the Vaginal Approach to Operative Gynecology. Johannesburg, USA: Witwatersrand University Press; 1965.p. 143.
10. Quinlan DK. Indications and contraindications. In: Sheth SS, Studd JW (Eds). Vaginal Hysterectomy, 2nd edition. London, UK: Martin Dunitz Ltd; 2002. pp. 7-14.
11. Zanagnolo V, Magrina JF. Carcinoma of the endometrium treated only by vaginal route. Best Pract Res Clin Obstet Gynaecol. 2011;25(2):239-45.
12. Faust G, Davies Q, Symonds P. Changes in the treatment of endometrial cancer. BJOG. 2010;117(9):1043-6.
13. Sheth SS. Newer perspectives. In: Sheth SS (Ed). Vaginal Hysterectomy, 2nd edition. New Delhi, India: Jaypee Brothers Medical Publishers (P) Ltd; 2014. pp. 225-34.
14. Sheth SS. Vaginal hysterectomy. Best Pract Res Clin Obstet Gynaecol. 2005;19(3):307-32.
15. Mariani A, Dowdy SC, Cliby WA, et al. Prospective assessment of lymphatic dissemination in endometrial cancer: a paradigm shift in surgical staging. Gynecol Oncol. 2008;109(1):11-8.
16. Creasman WT. Malignant tumors of the uterine corpus. In: Rock JA, Jones HW (Eds). TeLinde's Operative Gynecology, 9th edition. Philadelphia, PA, USA: Lippincott Williams & Wilkins; 2003. pp. 1445-86.

17. Morrow CP. Management of uterine neoplasia. In: Morrow CP, Curtin JP (Eds). Gynecologic Cancer Surgery, 1st edition. London, UK: Churchill Livingstone; 1996. pp. 569-625.
18. Hacker NF, Friedlander M. Uterine cancer. In: Berek JS, Hacker NF (Eds). Gynecology Oncology, 5th edition. Philadelphia, PA, USA: Lippincott Williams & Wilkins; 2010. pp. 396-442.
19. Arndt-Miercke H, Martin A, Briese V, et al. Transection of vaginal cuff is an independent prognostic factor in stage I endometrial cancer. Eur J Surg Oncol. 2008;34(2):241-6.
20. Stovall TG, Summitt RL Jr, Bran DF, et al. Outpatient vaginal hysterectomy: a pilot study. Obstet Gynecol. 1992;80(1):145-9.
21. Engh ME, Hauso W. Vaginal hysterectomy, an outpatient procedure. Acta Obstet Gynecol Scand. 2012;91(11):1293-9.
22. Paghdiwalla KP. Is vaginal hysterectomy a day care procedure? In: Sheth SS (Ed). Vaginal Hysterectomy, 2nd edition. New Delhi, India: Jaypee Brothers Medical Publishers (P) Ltd; 2014. pp. 207-9.

CASE 45: VH PLUS VAGINAL CUFF WITH BSO: POSTMENOPAUSAL BLEEDER WITH ENDOMETRIAL COMPLEX HYPERPLASIA WITH ATYPIA

Name: Mrs. X
Age: 78 years
Parity: 2 FTND (Full term normal delivery)
LD: 45 years back
Complains of (C/O): Postmenopausal vaginal bleeding
Last menstrual period (LMP): 28 years back

History of hysteroscopy plus D&C, 1 month back, giving diagnosis of complex endometrial hyperplasia with atypia. No malignancy.

Not obese. No H/O hypertension with diabetes.
Pelvic findings: Uterus was normal in size, healthy cervix with physiological descent and clear fornices.
Abdominopelvic sonography: It showed uterine dimensions 4.9 cm × 4.1 cm × 3 cm with ET of 4.2 mm and uterine volume 33 cm^3.
Diagnosis: Complex endometrial hyperplasia with atypia.
Operation: VH plus vaginal cuff with BSO and frozen HP study of uterus.
What deters/dissuades: If it turns out "cancer" of the endometrium and if myometrial wall is invaded to half or more.
Operation: VH started with vaginal cuff of 3 cm (Fig. 1) resected with uterus and proceeded to excise all the lateral connections of the uterus on one side and have the uterus with upper pedicle, tube, utero-ovarian and round ligament intact on the contralateral side. Traction on the free uterus facilitates cutting the round ligament as laterally as possible and perform salpingo-oophorectomy on the side of the intact upper pedicle. Soon after hysterectomy with unilateral salpingo-oophorectomy, uterus, tube and ovary were sent for frozen HP study of uterus to exclude uterine malignancy. Naked eye examination of the endometrial surface of cut open uterus appeared normal. No growth or polyp. This was followed by salpingo-oophorectomy of contralateral side (Age: 78 years) (Fig. 2).
Frozen HP study: It confirmed complex hyperplasia with atypia and no associated malignancy.

This proved beneficial as it spared patient from more invasive abdominal surgery.[1] In other words, the vaginal surgery proved adequate. This is not uncommon.

Had HP shown well-differentiated malignancy, it does not necessarily indicate lymphadenectomy, as long as MI is less than half or less than 50%[2,3] and therefore avoid need for opening of the abdomen or use of laparoscope.

Lymph node removal is required when malignancy has invaded half or more of the myometrial wall or there is

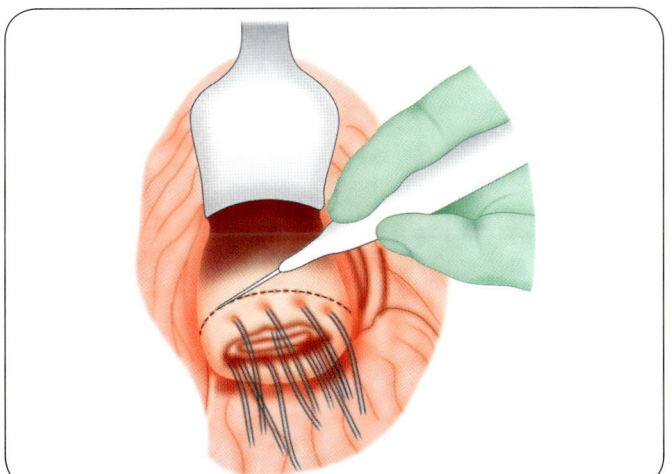

Fig. 1: The incision is continued anteriorly around the entire circumference of the vagina, taking care not to injure the bladder.
Source: In: Rock JA, Thompson JD (Eds). TeLinde's Operative Gynecology, 8th edition. Philadelphia, PA, USA: Lippincott-Raven Publishers; 1997. pp. 1413-99.

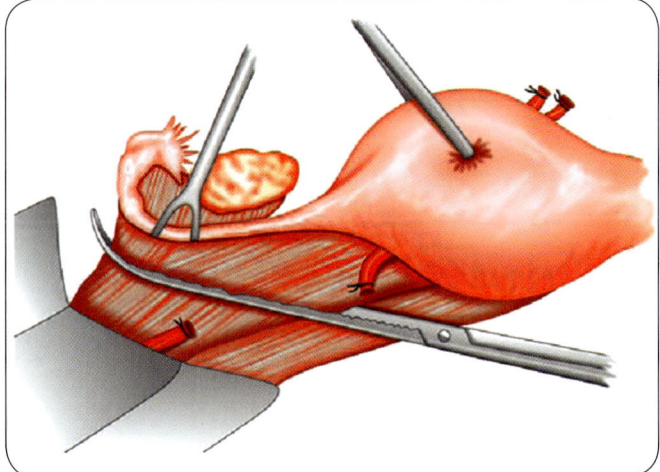

Fig. 2: A specially designed clamp is applied to infundibulopelvic ligament for a salpingo-oophorectomy.
Source: Adapted from "Sheth SS, Malpani AN. Technique of vaginal oophorectomy during vaginal hysterectomy. J Gynecol Surg. 1994; 10:197-202".

grade III/poorly differentiated carcinoma or it is clear cell "CA" or serous cell "CA" or carcinosarcoma, etc.

What inspired VH:
- Huge advantage of vaginal route over alternatives
- Elderly, 78 years old and diabetic
- Back up experience
- Taken as "Trial Vaginal Route". If malignancy indicated LNR, facilities for opening the abdomen or laparoscopic surgery were kept available.

Lymph node removal is not required, when malignancy has invaded half or less of the myometrial wall with well or moderately differentiated adenocarcinoma or endometrioid adenocarcinoma. LNR is contraindicated, if the woman is a high-risk patient and/or a candidate for high morbidity.[2,3]

Hemostasis was checked and closure done. Blood transfusion was not needed. Hospital stay was 2 days. Postoperative was uneventful with speedy recovery.

Histopathology: It showed uterus weighed 45 g. endometrial severe hyperplasia with atypia but no malignancy. Cervix, vaginal cuff, tubes and ovaries were normal.

LESSONS

- Advantage of the least invasive procedure
- Ideal to have a frozen HP facility for the just removed uterus.

Hence, for a woman with complex hyperplasia with atypia, VH with BSO and frozen HP of removed uterus is adequate treatment. Frozen HP of uterus will also guide the need for salpingo-oophorectomy or ovarian conservation, if the woman so desires. Important is foresight and prerequisites to be met with. However, one has to keep a small margin of safety as paraffin HP may upgrade and/or upstage the frozen HP report.[4]

To note:

World Health Organization (WHO) classifies into simple and complex hyperplasia and further each one of them with or without atypia:
- Simple hyperplasia with or without atypia
- Complex hyperplasia with or without atypia.

Kurman et al.[1] have shown that chance of developing malignancy is as follow:
- 8% for simple hyperplasia with atypia
- 29% for complex hyperplasia with atypia.

CASE 46: VH PLUS VAGINAL CUFF WITH BSO: POSTMENOPAUSAL BLEEDER WITH CORPUS CANCER SYNDROME FOR ENDOMETRIAL CANCER (CA)

Name: Mrs. X
Age: 75 years
Parity: 2 FTND
LD: 26 years
C/O: Postmenopausal vaginal bleeding for 8 weeks.
LMP: 20 years back

Obese [body mass index (BMI) 38, hypertensive and diabetic (corpus cancer syndrome).

Clinically 10 weeks size uterus with favorable descent of normal cervix to attempt VH. Fornices were clear.

Sonography: It showed enlarged uterus with volume of 150 cm^3, submucous small fibroid and ET of 30 mm.

She required hysteroscopy plus D & C or endometrial biopsy (EB) for endometrial HP study and further treatment accordingly. With corpus cancer syndrome, obesity, hypertension and diabetes, even if endometrial HP is benign, with a uterus of 10 weeks size, she needed hysterectomy, preferably. She preferred to have her uterus removed rather than go to the operation theater twice for surgery. This was discussed at length and she was well counseled.

Hence, it was decided to do VH and further depending on the frozen HP report of hysterectomized uterus.

Diagnosis: ?Polyp/?endometrial CA.
Operation: VH plus vaginal cuff with BSO.
What deters/dissuades: If "Cancer" of the endometrium is present and if myometrial wall is invaded half or more.

Vaginal hysterectomy with 3+ cm vaginal cuff[6-8] with BSO was performed.

Prefer to excise all the lateral connections of the uterus on one side (H/O unilateral salpingo-oophorectomy for ectopic pregnancy in the past) and have the uterus with intact other upper pedicle. Traction on free uterus on one side facilitated salpingo-oophorectomy of the contralateral side with intact upper pedicle.[9] Uterus, tube and ovary were sent for frozen HP study of uterus. Naked eye examination of cut open uterus revealed no growth or frank malignancy. Small area was unhealthy and congested.

Frozen HP report of the removed uterus was awaited to guide and/or dictate further treatment. Report was moderately differentiated endometrioid adenocarcinoma with MI of only 2 mm out of 23 mm (2.3 cm) (Fig. 1). Even after keeping safety margin from the final paraffin HP report,

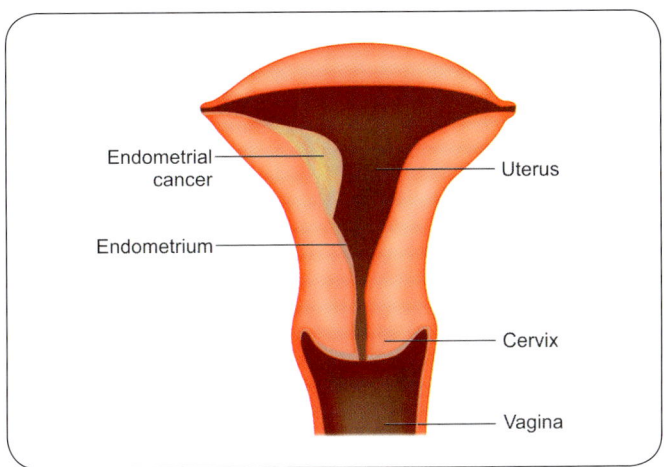

Fig. 1: Endometrial cancer.

the frozen section analysis should be applied by experienced pathologists and the possible predictive factors affecting a false diagnosis should carefully be taken into consideration.[10] Thus, the patient did not need LNR and further surgery.[5,6,11-17] Peritoneal fluid was collected again (earlier when POD was accessed) for cytology. After necessary checking including hemostasis of the vault, closure was done. Blood transfusion was not needed. Hospital stay was 2 days followed by speedy recovery.

Histopathology study: It showed uterine weight 168 g with leiomyoma and severe adenomyosis, negative vaginal cuff and normal adnexa: It confirmed endometrioid adenocarcinoma (2 mm out of 23 mm invasion), moderately differentiated with square metaplasia, adenoacanthoma of uterine corpus. Radiotherapist's opinion was taken for record and reassurance. The radiotherapist advised that there was no need for radiotherapy.

What inspired: Corpus CA syndrome, to reduce the risk and invasion.

LESSONS

- Spared from hysteroscopy plus D & C and morbidity from opening of the abdomen or laparoscopic surgery in an obese woman.[18]
- Vaginal hysterectomy would (a) eradicate disease containing uterus; (b) make the uterus available for frozen

HP to look for malignancy and if so, MI; (c) give an opportunity for concomitant BSO and (d) with frozen HP benign or malignancy but with MI less than half; generally no further treatment is required. Selectively the author often keeps a margin by lowering the limit to one-third from half, in case HP and paraffin HP study may differ.

Endometrial cancer may be:
- With myometrial wall invasion of half or more
- Poorly differentiated
- Clear cell or serous cell carcinoma or carcinosarcoma.

All of the above need LNR unless medically laparotomy or laparoscopic surgery is contraindicated because of high risk and resultant morbidity.

CASE 47: VH PLUS VAGINAL CUFF WITH BSO FOR ENDOMETRIAL CA

Name: Mrs. X
Age: 67 years
Parity: 4 FTND
C/O: Postmenopausal vaginal bleeding
LMP: 18 years back

Diabetic, hypertensive and not obese. Uterus 6 weeks size. Normal cervix with physiological descent to attempt VH. Fornices were clear. Sonography showed uterus volume 110 cm^3 with ET 22 mm. Tubes and ovaries were normal. H/O hysteroscopy plus D&C done with endometrial HP showing well-differentiated adenocarcinoma of endometrium. In other words, a case of endometrial "CA" for treatment.[19-25]

It was decided to take the vaginal route and proceed depending on the invasion of the myometrial wall from frozen HP study of the uterus.

Diagnosis: Well-differentiated adenocarcinoma of endometrium.

Operation: VH plus vaginal cuff with BSO.

What deters/dissuades: What about lymph node removal?

Vaginal cuff of 3 cm+ was prepared and VH done. Intraoperatively, the uterus along with one tube and ovary was sent for frozen HP study of uterus. Naked eye examination of the cut open uterus showed small ulcerated area in the endometrial lining, which was otherwise normal. Frozen HP study reported superficial MI by malignancy, less than one-fourth, 4 mm out of 21 mm (2.1 cm). In other words, frozen HP report favored nonremoval of lymph nodes, more so in a hypertensive and diabetic, a 67-year-old woman. This amounted to sparing her abdominal invasion from being opened or receiving five cuts for the laparoscopic surgery. Contralateral salpingo-oophorectomy was completed soon after sending the uterus for frozen HP study (Age: 67 years) as she desired removal of both ovaries.

Before closure obvious cystocele and rectocele were repaired to restore normalcy. Hemostasis was checked and vaginal closure done. Blood transfusion was not needed. Hospital stay was 2 days. She went home with an SR catheter for 2 more days because of anterior colporrhaphy and made an uneventful speedy recovery.

Histopathology: It showed uterine weight 136 g with normal wall except one area which revealed well-differentiated adenocarcinoma, invading 4 mm out of 21 mm of uterine wall.[5,19] Tubes, ovaries and vaginal cuff were negative.

Vaginal route offers a good look at cysto and rectoceles and if present, provides an opportunity to give additional benefit to the patient which is almost ignored at laparotomy or laparoscopic surgery.

What inspired: "IF" frozen favors nonremoval of lymph nodes.

LESSON

- Diabetic and hypertensive woman spared of opening of the abdomen or laparoscopic surgery and resultant morbidity.

CASE 48: VH PLUS VAGINAL CUFF WITH BSO: POSTMENOPAUSAL BLEEDER WITH CORPUS CANCER SYNDROME. FAILED "TRIAL VAGINAL ROUTE". ABDOMINAL SURGERY FOR LNR FOR ENDOMETRIAL CA

Name: Mrs. X
Age: 55 years
Parity: 3 FTND
LD: 27 years back
C/O: Postmenopausal vaginal bleeding
LMP: 15 years back

Obese (BMI: 33), hypertensive and diabetic (corpus cancer syndrome) (Fig. 1).

Clinically the uterus was 6 weeks in size, healthy cervix with favorable descent to attempt VH and clear fornices.

Sonography: It showed uterine dimensions of 6 cm × 5.3 cm × 4.5 cm with 75 cm^3 volume, cervical polyp of 3 cm × 1.5 cm with ET of 17 mm and normal ovaries.

No past H/O hysteroscopy or D & C.

Diagnosis: ?Endometrial hyperplasia, ?cancer.

Operation: VH plus vaginal cuff with BSO → Frozen HP → Endometrioid carcinoma with invasion of 1.3 cm/2.2 cm → Abdominally LNR, etc.

What deters/dissuades VH: If endometrial "CA" with 50% or more MI.

Vaginal cuff plus VH with one-sided salpingo-oophorectomy was performed. On naked eye examination, the cut uterus showed frank carcinomatous growth in the upper part of the uterus. Rest of the uterus and cervix along with the tubes and ovaries appeared normal. The uterus with one tube and ovary was sent for frozen section HP of the uterus. The patient was keen to have her ovaries removed. Meanwhile, contralateral salpingo-oophorectomy was completed. Frozen section HP reported moderately differentiated endometrioid carcinoma with invasion of 1.3 cm out of 2.2 cm uterine wall plus endocervix and cervical stroma invasion.[2,3,6] The tubes, ovaries and vaginal cuff were free of malignancy. Peritoneal fluid and lavage fluid was taken for cytology before vaginal closure. As MI was more than half, it was decided to perform LNR and more, if required. Therefore with Pfannenstiel's incision, the abdomen was opened for removal of bilateral pelvic chain of lymph nodes.[13,17,19] They were removed as per the routine. The aortic bifurcation and the inferior vena caval area were carefully inspected and found to be clear or

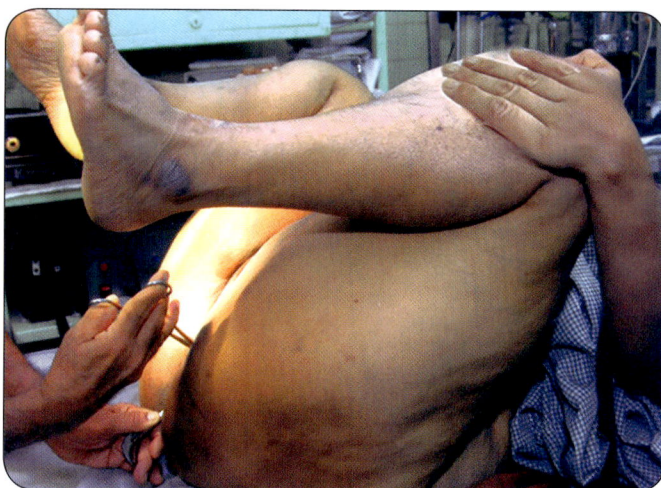

Fig. 1: The patient's both hands are keeping her both feet apart and thus providing clear view of the vulva vaginal area and required speculum examination.
Source: In: Sheth SS (Ed). Vaginal Hysterectomy, 2nd edition. New Delhi, India: Jaypee Brothers Medical Publishers (P) Ltd; 2014. pp. 225-34.

normal. The liver was normal. After full inspection, peritoneal fluid was taken for cytology, hemostasis was checked and abdominal closure completed.

Blood loss was minimal. Blood transfusion was not needed. Hospital stay was 5 days. Postoperative period was uneventful with a speedy recovery.

Histopathology report: The uterus weighed 96 g showed endometrioid adenocarcinoma, moderately differentiated with MI of 1.4 cm out of 2.2 cm of myometrial wall plus endocervix and cervical stromal invasion. Lymphovascular invasion was negative. Lymph nodes were negative for malignancy. The tubes, ovaries and vaginal cuff were normal.

She was referred to the radiotherapy and chemotherapy units for opinion and further treatment.

The vaginal route was chosen for hysterectomy plus vaginal cuff with BSO, hoping that frozen HP may indicate nonremoval of the lymph nodes as it happens often. Hypertension, diabetes and obesity, strengthened this need to spare abdominal invasion. Obviously in performing VH, it is the frozen section HP report that dictates further treatment. No doubt, one may insist on magnetic resonance imaging (MRI) for decision making, i.e. MRI showing MI and accordingly the approach can be vaginal OR abdominal. However, unfortunately, in practice I have come across occasions when MRI reports have been grossly wrong or misused. A morbidly obese woman with hypertension and diabetes undergoing abdominal surgery because of MRI showing more than half thickness invasion and later frozen HP of uterus showing less than one-third MI, is not uncommon. Therefore, it is not always easy to depend solely on the MRI.

What inspired: If for a patient with corpus cancer syndrome, surgical invasion could be reduced!

LESSON

- Always be ready to open the abdomen and treat fully, if and when required.

CASE 49: VH PLUS VAGINAL CUFF WITH BSO FOR ENDOMETRIAL COMPLEX HYPERPLASIA WITH ATYPIA. CORPUS CA SYNDROME PLUS A HISTORY OF CARDIAC BYPASS

Name: Mrs. X
Age: 61 years
Parity: 2 FTND
LMP: 12 years back
C/O: Recurrent postmenopausal vaginal bleeding, pain in lower abdomen with dribble of urine on straining.
H/O: Cardiac bypass and H/O having 3 stents.

Morbidly obese (BMI: 41),[18,26-31] hypertensive, diabetic (corpus cancer syndrome) and with hypothyroidism.

Clinically uterus was 6 weeks size with small cervical polyp and favorable cervix to attempt VH (Fig. 1).

Sonography: It revealed uterus with 7.3 cm × 4.8 cm × 4.5 cm dimensions, volume 85 cm³ with 2 cm fibroid, ET of 8 mm and normal ovaries.
Diagnosis: ?Endometrial hyperplasia, ?Endometrial cancer.
Operation: VH plus vaginal cuff with BSO.
What deters/dissuades: If malignant and myometrial involvement is half or more.

Patient was fully counseled with pros and cons discussed at length. VH with vaginal cuff of 3 cm with unilateral salpingo-oophorectomy was done and promptly sent for frozen HP study of uterus. Naked eye examination of cut open uterus showed normal endometrium and uterine walls. Meanwhile, remaining contralateral salpingo-oophorectomy was completed. Frozen HP reported endometrial complex hyperplasia with atypia[1] plus simple polyp—all without malignancy. Hemostasis was checked and vaginal closure done. Blood transfusion was not needed.

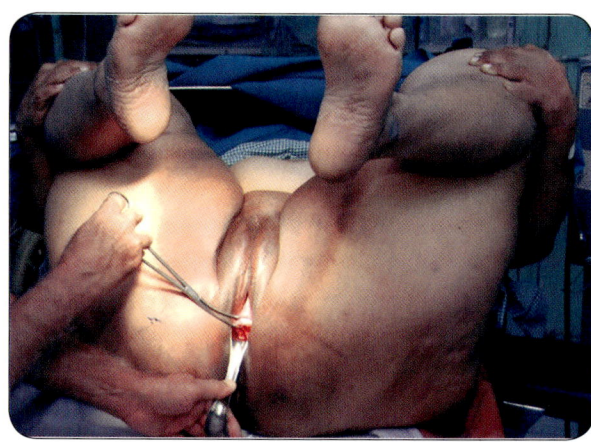

Fig. 1: Superflexion position. The patient's hands keep both feet apart and thus provide a clear view of the vulva and vaginal area.[31]

Hospital stay was 2 days followed by an uneventful speedy recovery.

Paraffin HP confirmed the frozen HP report of no malignancy and complex hyperplasia with atypia. Uterus weighed 110 g with normal tubes and ovaries.

What inspired: If for a corpus cancer syndrome patient, surgical invasion could be reduced!

LESSON

- Vaginal route spared high risk morbidly obese woman of greater invasion and morbidity from abdominal access via laparotomy or laparoscopy.

CASE 50: VH PLUS VAGINAL CUFF WITH BSO FOR WELL-DIFFERENTIATED ENDOMETRIAL ADENOCARCINOMA

Name: Mrs. X
Age: 60 years
Parity: 1 FTND
C/O: Recurrent postmenopausal vaginal bleeding.
LMP: 2 years back.
She was referred with H/O Hysteroscopy plus dilation and curettage (D&C) and diagnosis of well-differentiated endometrioid adenocarcinoma.
Obese (BMI 43),[18,26-30] diabetic and nonhypertensive.
Clinically uterus 12 weeks size, healthy cervix with physiological descent and clear fornices.
Sonography: It revealed uterine volume of 280 cm^3, endometrial thickness 18 mm and normal pelvic findings.
Management was discussed at length; pros and cons explained including sparing opening of the abdomen or need to open it.
Diagnosis: Well-differentiated endometrioid adenocarcinoma.
Operation: VH plus vaginal cuff with BSO.
What deters/dissuades: If myometrial wall is invaded to half or more.

VH with vaginal cuff and unilateral salpingo-oophorectomy was performed without difficulty. She needed extra traction on uterus and lateral wall retraction for completion of hysterectomy. Much depended on frozen HP report of myometrial invasion of hysterectomized uterus sent for the study. Meanwhile, contralateral salpingo-oophorectomy was completed. Frozen HP reported 5 mm invasion out of 24 mm of myometrial thickness.[2,6,19,25] This ruled out lymph node removal (LNR) and therefore, laparotomy or laparoscopic surgery.[11,13-14] Hemostasis was checked and vaginal closure done. Blood transfusion was not needed. Hospital stay was 2 days followed by an uneventful speedy recovery.

What inspired: If Frozen HP reports in favor of non removal of lymph nodes, i.e. abdominal access will be spared.

LESSONS

- Obese and diabetic with endometrial CA easily spared from opening of the abdomen.
- Vaginal hysterectomy plus cuff with BSO proved adequate.

CASE 51: VH PLUS VAGINAL CUFF WITH BSO: POSTMENOPAUSAL BLEEDER WITH ENDOMETRIAL CA WITH HISTORY OF TWO CAESAREAN SECTIONS FOLLOWED BY INCISIONAL HERNIA REPAIR

Name: Mrs. X
Age: 60 years
Parity: 2 FTCS (H/O: Abdominal hernioplasty with mesh for incisional hernia).
  No H/O normal delivery (ND).
C/O: Bleeding per vaginam since 3 months.
LMP: 12 years back.
  No H/O hysteroscopy plus D & C or EB
  Obese (BMI: 38).[18,26-31] Hypertensive and nondiabetic.
  Uterus was normal size with ET 18 mm on sonography. Other abdominopelvic findings were normal.
  Decided to perform VH and get guided by frozen HP report of the uterus.
Diagnosis: ?Endometrial hyperplasia/?cancer.
Operation: VH plus vaginal cuff with BSO → Frozen HP → Endometrial "CA" (3 mm/18 mm) → No further surgery.
What deters/dissuades: If "cancer" and if it invades half or more of the uterine or myometrial wall.
Operation: VH with 3 cm vaginal cuff done. Bladder separated with help of uterocervical-broad ligament space (Fig. 1). Soon after hysterectomy along with unilateral salpingo-oophorectomy, uterus, tube and ovary were sent for frozen HP study of uterus to exclude endometrial malignancy. Naked eye examination of the cut open uterus showed normal endometrium except tiny area appearing vascular and unhealthy. Prefer to excise all the lateral connections of the uterus on one side and have the uterus with the upper pedicle, tube, utero-ovarian and round ligaments intact on the contralateral side. Meanwhile traction on the free uterus from one side facilitates salpingo-oophorectomy of the contralateral side with the intact upper pedicle.
  Frozen HP reported severe atypia with complex hyperplasia plus focal endometrial "CA", invading 3 mm depth out of 18 mm of myometrial wall. Focal endometrioid adenocarcinoma was moderately differentiated with minimal invasion of myometrial wall. She needed no further surgery.[3,6,11,13,32,33]
  Thus, major invasion as well as resulting morbidity from LNR was spared by VH plus vaginal cuff with BSO.

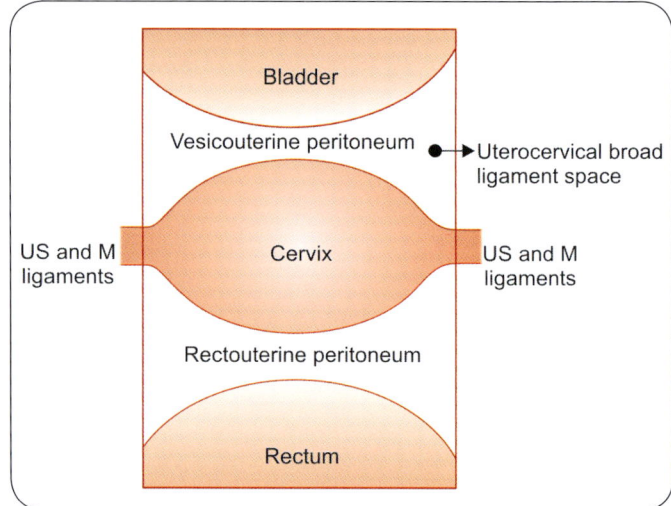

Fig. 1: This figure distinctly shows the space between bladder and cervix or cervicouterine surface, which is much more under lateral one-fifth of bladder when compared with central three-fifths of bladder. *Source*: In: Sheth SS (Ed). Vaginal Hysterectomy, 2nd edition. New Delhi, India: Jaypee Brothers Medical Publishers (P) Ltd; 2014. pp. 31-50.

Abdominal access would not have been easy with an H/O two lower segment caesarean sections (LSCS) and an incisional hernia repair in the past.[20,34-37]
  Hemostasis was checked and vaginal closure done. Blood transfusion was not needed. Hospital stay was 2 days, followed by speedy recovery.
Histopathology: It showed uterus weighed 35 g with normal endometrium except in small area showing endometrioid adenocarcinoma, moderately differentiated with 5 mm invasion out of 18 mm of myometrial wall. Tubes, ovaries and vaginal cuff were normal.
What inspired: Contraindicated abdominal route for hysterectomy.[35]

LESSON

- Caesarean sections followed by incisional hernia repair did not deter but added flavor and saved opening of the abdomen for the fourth time.

CASE 52: VH PLUS VAGINAL CUFF WITH BSO PLUS LAPAROSCOPIC CHOLECYSTECTOMY FOR POSTMENOPAUSAL BLEEDER WITH MULTIPLE GALLSTONES

Name: Mrs. X
Age: 54 years
Parity: 2 FTCS
LD: 29 years back
C/O: Postmenopausal vaginal bleeding.
LMP: 3 years back.

Morbidly obese (BMI: 47),[18,26-31] hypertensive and non-diabetic with symptomatic gallstones. Clinically uterus 8 weeks size. Cervix with physiological descent and clear fornices. Sonography showed uterine volume of 160 cm³, ET of 11 mm with normal pelvic findings and gallbladder showed multiple stones (Fig. 1).

Needed "laparoscopic" cholecystectomy plus hysteroscopy plus D&C, HP study and later depending on HP report. However, after necessary counseling, she preferred to have laparoscopic cholecystectomy and VH at one sitting and further management depending on the frozen HP report of hysterectomized uterus. Therefore, it was decided to have cholecystectomy and hysterectomy at one sitting.[38-47]

Diagnosis: ?Endometrial hyperplasia, ?malignancy plus gallbladder calculi.

Operation: Laparoscopic cholecystectomy followed by VH plus vaginal cuff with BSO.

What deters/dissuades: If endometrial "CA" and if it invades half or more of myometrial wall.

First laparoscopic cholecystectomy was performed (Fig. 1) by a surgeon Dr T Udwadia followed by a change of patient's position to lithotomy and then doing vaginal hysterectomy. Uterocervical-broad ligament space was helpful to get an access to the vesicouterine peritoneum as she had a H/O two caesarean sections in past (Fig. 2). VH with BSO was completed. Naked eye examination showed endometrium, uterine cavity and uterus normal. Uterus with one tube and ovary sent for frozen HP study. Frozen HP study of hysterectomized uterus reported, endometrial complex hyperplasia without atypia and no malignancy. No further surgery was required.

Hemostasis was checked and vaginal closure done. Blood transfusion was not needed. Hospital stay was 2 days followed by an uneventful speedy recovery.

Histopathology: It confirmed complex hyperplasia, no atypia, adenomyosis with normal tubes and ovaries. No malignancy. Uterus weighed 190 g. Gallbladder showed chronic cholecystitis with multiple stones.

This gave a sigh of relief as morbidly obese woman was spared of laparotomy or 4 or 5 additional abdominal holes, much greater invasion as well as resultant morbidity. She got an advantage of laparoscopic cholecystectomy and hysterectomy at one session/sitting, i.e. killing two birds with one stone. Something gratifying!

What inspired: Attempt to reduce the invasion.

LESSONS

- VH plus cuff with BSO and laparoscopic cholecystectomy performed at one surgical session
- H/O caesarean sections in the past and morbid obesity added flavor.

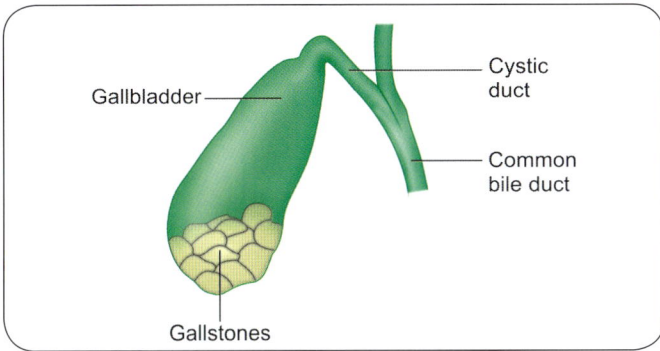

Fig. 1: Gallbladder with stones.

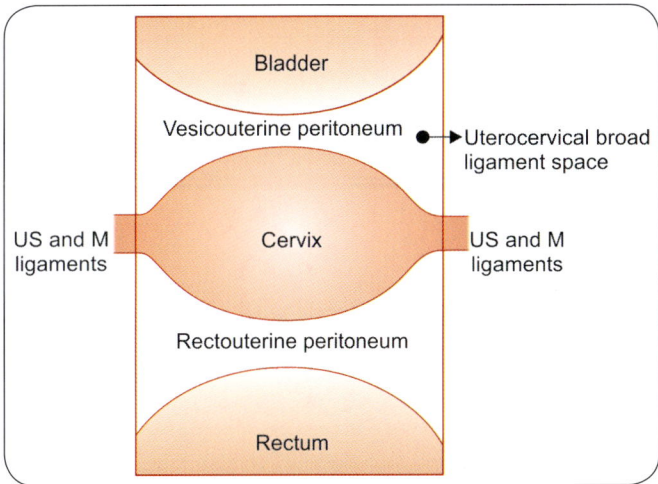

Fig. 2: This figure distinctly shows the space between bladder and cervix or cervicouterine surface, which is much more under lateral one-fifth of bladder when compared with central three-fifths of bladder.
Source: In: Sheth SS (Ed). Vaginal Hysterectomy, 2nd edition. New Delhi, India: Jaypee Brothers Medical Publishers (P) Ltd; 2014. pp. 31-50.

CASE 53: LAPAROSCOPIC CHOLECYSTECTOMY AND VH PLUS VAGINAL CUFF WITH BSO: "FAILED TRIAL VAGINAL ROUTE CASE" ABDOMINAL LNR FOR ENDOMETRIAL CA

Name: Mrs. X
Age: 78 years
Parity: 5 FTND
LD: 38 years back
C/O: Postmenopausal vaginal bleeding.
LMP: 30 years back.

H/O hysteroscopy plus D&C with HP showing endometrioid "CA" plus abdominal sonography showing symptomatic multiple gallstones.

Not obese but hypertensive and diabetic.

Clinically normal size uterus. Healthy cervix with favorable descent to attempt vaginal hysterectomy. Fornices were clear. Sonography showed uterus 6 cm × 3.8 cm × 3.7 cm with volume of 46 cm^3. ET 13 mm, ovaries not seen.

Diagnosis: Well-differentiated endometrioid CA, plus cholecystitis due to multiple gallstones. Taken as "Trial Vaginal Route Case".

Operation: Laparoscopic cholecystectomy + VH with vaginal cuff plus BSO → Failed "Trial Vaginal Route" (MI 8 mm out of 14 mm) → Abdominal LNR, etc.

What deters/dissuades: If myometrial wall is invaded to half or more.

She needed laparoscopic cholecystectomy plus management of endometrioid adenocarcinoma. Full treatment depended on frozen HP of uterus showing degree of MI. First laparoscopic cholecystectomy was performed by Dr Shirish K Bhansali, followed by change in position to lithotomy for VH with salpingo-oophorectomy.[39,40,46] First vaginal cuff of 3–4 cm is prepared and hysterectomy with unilateral salpingo-oophorectomy performed vaginally without any difficulty. Uterus with tube and ovary sent for frozen HP of uterus. Naked eye examination of cut open uterus showed small unhealthy, cancerous looking area in uterine body. Meanwhile, remaining, contralateral salpingo-oophorectomy completed followed by much required AP repair. Frozen HP showed 8 mm involvement of the myometrium out of 14 mm, i.e. more than half or 50% invasion[2] (Fig. 1). Thus, she needed lymph nodes removal, i.e. abdominal approach.[6,11,13,19] Hemostasis was checked and vaginal closure done after taking fluid for cytology. She was then taken for laparotomy for LNR. Abdomen opened with Pfannenstiel's incision and bilateral pelvic node removal done. More than 12 lymph nodes with fibro-fatty tissue removed. Aortic, inferior vena cava (IVC) area was clear with normal liver. After checking hemostasis, etc. abdomen was closed in layers. Blood transfusion was not needed. Hospital stay was 5 days followed by an uneventful speedy recovery.

Later, paraffin HP reported endometrioid adenocarcinoma, International Federation of Gynecology and Obstetrics (FIGO) Grade II, moderately differentiated. 8 mm out of 14 mm myometrial wall was invaded. Lymphovascular invasion present with all the lymph nodes negative. Uterus normal size, weighed 65 g. Cervix, vaginal cuff margins, tubes and ovaries were negative. Chronic cholecystitis with multiple gallstones.

Had huge advantage of combining gallbladder surgery—laparoscopic cholecystectomy, which was first performed.[42,46] Earlier, she was fully assessed to be fit for both operations, including abdominal, if it became necessary.

If gynecologist is used to doing LNR, it becomes easy and handy to perform VH and go by frozen HP report. Do not have to arrange for standby oncosurgeon or have last minute hassle.

What inspired: To reduce the invasion, if possible.

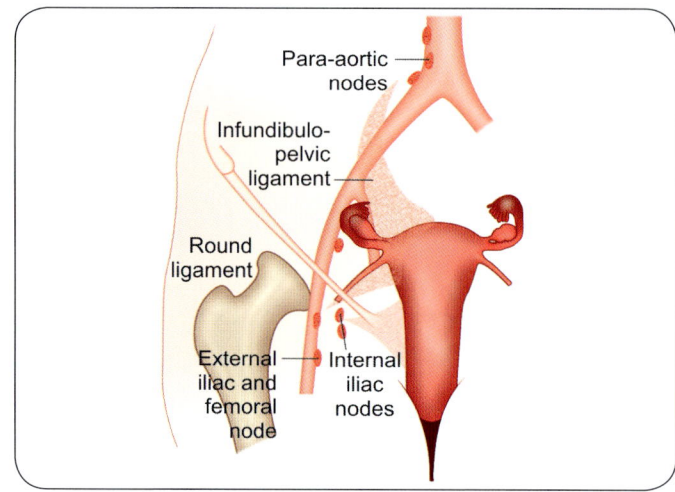

Fig. 1: Lymphatic pathways of tumor spread of endometrial carcinoma to pelvic and extra-pelvic nodes.[1]

LESSON

- Be prepared for the abdominal approach for LNR plus.

REFERENCES

1. Kurman RJ, Kaminski PF, Norris HJ. The behavior of endometrial hyperplasia. A long-term study of "untreated" hyperplasia in 170 patients. Cancer. 1985;56(2):403-12.
2. Pecorelli S. Revised FIGO staging for carcinoma of the vulva, cervix, and endometrium. Int J Gynecol Obstet. 2009;105(2):103-4.
3. Jones HW 3rd. New developments in the surgical management of early endometrial cancer. Obstet Gynecol. 2009;114(1):2-3.
4. Kumar S, Bandyopadhyay S, Semaan A, et al. The role of frozen section in surgical staging of low risk endometrial cancer. PLoS One. 2011;6(9):e21912.
5. Sheth SS, Paghdiwalla KP, Hajari AR. Vaginal route: a gynaecological route for much more than hysterectomy. Best Pract Res Clin Obstet Gynaecol. 2011;25(2):115-32.
6. Zanagnolo V, Magrina JF. Carcinoma of the endometrium treated only by vaginal route. Best Pract Res Clin Obstet Gynaecol. 2011;25(2):239-45.
7. Arndt-Miercke H, Martin A, Briese V, et al. Transection of vaginal cuff is an independent prognostic factor in stage I endometrial cancer. Eur J Surg Oncol. 2008;34(2):241-6.
8. Mariani A, Dowdy SC, Cliby WA, et al. Prospective assessment of lymphatic dissemination in endometrial cancer: a paradigm shift in surgical staging. Gynecol Oncol. 2008;109(1):11-8.
9. Sheth SS. Adnexectomy for benign pathology at vaginal hysterectomy without laparoscopic assistance. BJOG. 2002;109(12):1401-5.
10. Gultekin E, Gultekin OE, Cingillioglu B, et al. The value of frozen section evaluation in the management of borderline ovarian tumors. J Cancer Res Ther. 2011;7(4):416-20.
11. The writing committee on behalf of the ASTEC study group. Efficacy of systematic pelvic lymphadenectomy in endometrial cancer (MRC ASTEC trial): A randomised study. Lancet. 2009;373(9658):125-36.
12. Hacker NF, Friedlander M. Uterine cancer. In: Berek JS, Hacker NF (Eds). Gynecology Oncology, 5th edition. Philadelphia, PA, USA: Lippincott Williams & Wilkins; 2010. pp. 396-442.
13. Benedetti Panici P, Basile S, Maneschi F, et al. Systematic pelvic lymphadenectomy vs. no lymphadenectomy in early-stage endometrial carcinoma: randomized clinical trial. J Natl Cancer Inst. 2008;100(23):1707-16.
14. Berretta R, Merisio C, Melpignano M, et al. Vaginal versus abdominal hysterectomy in endometrial cancer: a retrospective study in a selective population. Int J Gynecol Cancer. 2008;18(4):797-802.
15. Bloss JD, Berman ML, Bloss LP, et al. Use of vaginal hysterectomy for the management of stage I endometrial cancer in the medically compromised patient. Gynecol Oncol. 1991;40(1):74-7.
16. Chan JK, Lin YG, Monk BJ, et al. Vaginal hysterectomy as primary treatment of endometrial cancer in medically compromised women. Obstet Gynecol. 2001;97(5 Pt 1):707-11.
17. Magrina JF, Mutone NF, Weaver AL, et al. Laparoscopic lymphadenectomy and vaginal or laparoscopic hysterectomy with bilateral salpingo-oophorectomy for endometrial cancer: morbidity and survival. Am J Obstet Gynecol. 1999;181(2):376-81.
18. Sheth SS. Vaginal hysterectomy as primary route for morbidly obese women. Acta Obstet Gynecol Scand. 2010;89(7):971-4.
19. Zanagnolo V, Magrina JF. Vaginal hysterectomy for carcinoma of the endometrium. In: Sheth SS (Ed). Vaginal Hysterectomy, 2nd edition. New Delhi, India: Jaypee Brothers Medical Publishers (P) Ltd; 2014. pp. 216-24.
20. Sheth SS. Vaginal or abdominal hysterectomy? In: Sheth SS (Ed). Vaginal Hysterectomy, 2nd edition. New Delhi, India: Jaypee Brothers Medical Publishers (P) Ltd; 2014. pp. 273-93.
21. Ingiulla W, Cosmi EV. Vaginal hysterectomy for the treatment of cancer of the corpus uteri. Am J Obstet Gynecol. 1968;100(4):541-3.
22. Krige CF. Vaginal hysterectomy and genital prolapse repair. A contribution to the vaginal approach to operative gynecology. Johannesburg, USA: Witwatersrand University Press; 1965. p. 143.
23. Quinlan DK. Indications and contraindications. In: Sheth SS, Studd JW (Eds). Vaginal Hysterectomy. London, UK: Martin Dunitz Ltd; 2002. pp. 7-14.
24. Faust G, Davies Q, Symonds P. Changes in the treatment of endometrial cancer. BJOG. 2010;117(9):1043-6.
25. Massi G, Savino L, Susini T. Vaginal hysterectomy versus abdominal hysterectomy for the treatment of stage I endometrial adenocarcinoma. Am J Obstet Gynecol. 1996;174(4):1320-6.
26. Pitkin RM. Abdominal hysterectomy in obese women. Surg Gynecol Obstet. 1976;142(4):532-6.
27. Foley K, Lee RB. Surgical complications of obese patients with endometrial carcinoma. Gynecol Oncol. 1990;39(2):171-4.
28. Rafii A, Samain E, Levardon M, et al. Vaginal hysterectomy for benign disorders in obese women: a prospective study. BJOG. 2005;112(2):223-7.
29. Lean ME. Prognosis in obesity. BMJ. 2005;330(7504):1339-40.
30. Liston WA, Alexander C. Operating on the obese woman. In: Hillard T (Ed). The Yearbook of Obstetrics and Gynaecology, Volume 12. London, UK: RCOG Press; 2008. pp. 206-9.
31. Sheth SS. Super flexion position for difficult speculum examination. Int J Gynaecol Obstet. 2013;121(1):92-3.
32. Creasman WT. Malignant tumors of the uterine corpus. In: Rock JA, Jones HW (Eds). TeLinde's Operative Gynecology, 9th edition. Philadelphia, PA, USA: Lippincott Williams & Wilkins; 2003. pp. 1445-86.
33. Morrow CP. Management of uterine neoplasia. In: Morrow CP, Curtin JP (Eds). Gynecologic Cancer Surgery, 1st edition. London, UK: Churchill Livingstone; 1996. pp. 569-625.
34. Sheth SS. Vaginal hysterectomy. In: Studd J (Ed). Progress in Obstetrics and Gynecology, 10th edition. London, UK: Churchill Livingstone; 1993. pp. 317-40.

35. Sheth SS. Contraindicated abdominal route. In: Sheth SS (Ed). Vaginal Hysterectomy, 2nd edition. New Delhi, India: Jaypee Brothers Medical Publishers (P) Ltd; 2014. pp. 123-8.
36. Sheth SS, Shah VM. Hysterectomy after previous abdominopelvic surgery. In: Sheth SS (Ed). Vaginal Hysterectomy, 2nd edition. New Delhi, India: Jaypee Brothers Medical Publishers (P) Ltd; 2014. pp. 110-5.
37. Sheth SS, Paghdiwalla KP. Do we need the laparoscopic route? J Obstet Gynaecol India. 2001;51:25-30.
38. Pratt JH, O'Leary JA, Symmonds RE. Combined cholecystectomy and hysterectomy: a study of 95 cases. Mayo Clin Proc. 1967;42(9):529-35.
39. Sheth SS, Bhansali SK, Goyal MV, et al. Cholecystectomy and hysterectomy: a least invasive approach. J Gynecol Surg. 1997;13:181-5.
40. Murray JM, Glistrap LC 3rd, Massey FM. Cholecystectomy and abdominal hysterectomy. JAMA. 1980;244(20):2305-6.
41. Widdison AL. A systematic review of the effectiveness and safety of laparoscopic cholecystectomy. Ann R Coll Surg Eng. 1996;78(5):476.
42. Bhansali SK, Sheth SS. Associated non-gynecological surgery. In: Sheth SS, Studd JW (Eds). Vaginal Hysterectomy, 2nd edition. London, UK: Martin Dunitz Ltd; 2002. pp. 237-42.
43. Wadhwa A, Chowbey PK, Sharma A, et al. Combined procedures in laparoscopic surgery. Surg Laparosc Endosc Percutan Tech. 2003;13(6):382-6.
44. Sheth SS. Vaginal hysterectomy. Best Pract Res Clin Obstet Gynaecol. 2005;19(3):307-32.
45. Udwadia TE. Laparoscopic Cholecystectomy, 1st edition. Bombay, India: Oxford University Press; 1991.
46. Udwadia TE, Sheth SS. Associated non-gynecological surgery. In: Sheth SS (Ed). Vaginal Hysterectomy, 2nd edition. New Delhi, India: Jaypee Brothers Medical Publishers (P) Ltd; 2014. pp. 243-7.
47. Adanu RM, Hammoud MM. Contemporary issues in women's health. Int J Obstet Gynecol. 2010;109:3-4.

Section 6

FAILED TRIAL VAGINAL HYSTERECTOMY/ TRIAL VAGINAL ROUTE

> *"We do not, what we ought to
> What we ought not, we do
> And then lean upon a thought that chance will bring us through."*
> —Matthew Arnold

CASES

Dr Shirish S Sheth

Case 54: Undiagnosed Uteroabdominal Band
Case 55: Uterocervical Adhesions with Abdominal Wall
Case 56: Diminished "Uterus-free" Space (Altered Uterocervical Angle)
Case 57: Ovarian Endometriosis with Positive "Dimple Sign"
Case 58: Large-sized Uterus
Case 59: Ovarian Malignancy

Dr Seth Finkelstein

Case 60: Uterine Bulk Impedes Descent
Case 61: Extensive Adhesions from PID (Pelvic Inflammatory Disease) Limits Descent for VH
Case 62: Unanticipated Uterine Adhesions to Abdominal Wall-1
Case 63: Unanticipated Uterine Adhesions to Abdominal Wall-2
Case 64: Unanticipated Uterine Adhesions to Abdominal Wall-3
Case 65: Parasitic Myoma and Inaccessible Adnexa Leads to Laparoscopic Completion of VH

CASE 54: UNDIAGNOSED UTEROABDOMINAL BAND

Name: Mrs. X
Age: 40 years
Parity: 1 FTCS
Complains of (C/O): Heavy, painful menses and abdominal pain.

Clinically uterus was 12 weeks size and mobile. Normal cervix with physiological descent and clear fornices.
Sonography: Normal abdominopelvic findings. Uterus volume 250 cm³ with normal adnexa. However, an experienced sonologist Dr Darshana Kshirsagar from NM Medical Center, Mumbai, India, had put it abdominal wall adhesions, i.e. between uterus and abdominal wall.[1,2] The patient was taken as "trial vaginal hysterectomy (VH) case".[3,4]

Cervix with physiological descent favored VH as findings were the same under anesthesia with a negative "cervicofundal" sign.
Diagnosis: Severe adenomyosis.
Operation: Failed "Trial VH", Laparoscopic adhesiolysis of "band" followed by laparoscopically-assisted vaginal hysterectomy (LAVH).
What deters/dissuades VH: If adhesions are present.

Access to vesicouterine peritoneum was with the help of uterocervical-broad ligament space.[5,6] After uterine vessels were secured, cervix was bisected to debulk the uterus as much as possible. Despite almost reaching close to the round ligaments, there was no uterine descent with upright posterior uterine wall and no more lateral connections available to access. Respecting sonographic doubt, trial was accepted as "failed" and laparoscopy done to look for adhesions. There was a small 2 cm thick band, binding the upper uterine body with the abdominal wall, similar to shown in Figures 1A and B. Laparoscopically band was cut to release the uterus and complete the hysterectomy vaginally. Adhesions did not bind the uterocervical surface and lower abdominal wall surface but two were bound by a "band" of adhesion.

Healthy ovaries were preserved and raw areas cauterized. Hemostasis was confirmed and closure done. Blood transfusion was not needed. Hospital stay was 3 days with a speedy recovery.
Histopathology (HP): It showed uterus weighed 290 g with severe adenomyosis. No malignancy.

Respecting sonographic hint "trial VH" was attempted and later it proved worth as looking inside the peritoneal cavity with a laparoscope gave the cause of hindrance.

In fact, it was a learning experience for the future as mere band differs from surface-to-surface adhesions between the abdominal wall and uterocervical surface that follow caesarean section(s) in the past and give a positive "cervicofundal" sign.[1]
What inspired: Normal cervical descent.

LESSON

- To respect reliable sonography findings, though in this case, it was a "band" and not described adhesions.[1,2]

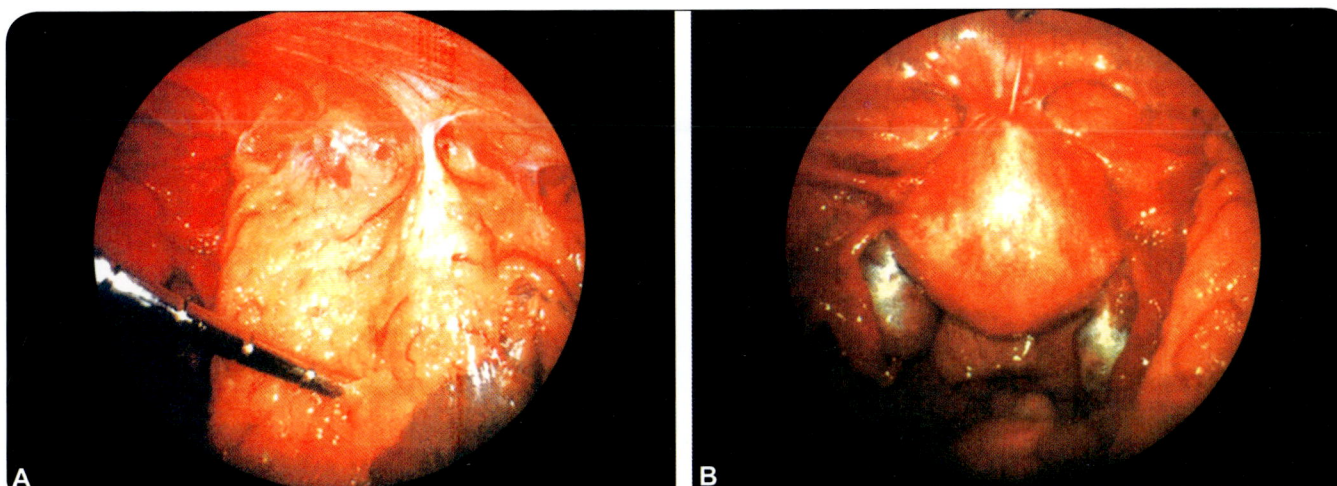

Figs. 1A and B: (A) Preoperative view of the pelvis. It shows band hold the uterus and the same free uterus after adhesiolysis in (B)
Source: In: Sutton C, Diamond MP (Eds). Endoscopic Surgery for Gynecologists, 2nd edition. London, UK: WB Saunders; 1998. pp. 300-7.

CASE 55: UTEROCERVICAL ADHESIONS WITH ABDOMINAL WALL

Name: Mrs. X
Age: 48 years
Parity: 2 FTCS
LD: 15 years back
C/O: Heavy menses

Clinically uterine size could not be made out. Uterine mobility was absent. Cervix was felt with difficulty, high up and anteriorly close to the pubic symphysis. Fornices were clear.

Sonography and magnetic resonance imaging (MRI) revealed uterine volume 110 cm^3 with fundus almost near the umbilicus. In other words, 6 weeks size uterus with fundus at too high level. Tubes and ovaries were normal.

Diagnosis: Uterine adenomyosis. Adhesions with abdominal wall[1,2,7] (This was the earliest case and therefore a query from the sonologist).

Operation: Failed "trial VH"[3,4] followed by abdominal hysterectomy.

What deters/dissuades: Possible trauma to bladder or more.

Under anesthesia, the cervix was barely seen and vulsellum was applied with difficulty. Posterior vaginal wall was pulled up and stretched. When traction was applied to the cervix, it caused dimpling in the lower abdominal wall, signaling that the uterus is likely to be adherent to the abdominal wall.[1] Anteriorly for bladder separation, getting uterocervical-broad ligament space, there was no plane of cleavage. In fact, there was extra oozing. Therefore, it was decided to give up and open the abdomen. After opening the abdomen there were dense adhesions from the uterocervical surface and bladder to the lower abdominal wall. Uterine fundus was free but disproportionately high up near the umbilicus for the size of uterus with elongated cervix.[1] Adhesions were carefully separated to free the uterus and bladder and hysterectomy was completed. Hemostasis was checked and vaginal closure done. Blood transfusion was not needed. Hospital stay was 5 days with an uneventful recovery (Figs. 1 to 5).

Histopathology: It showed severe adenomyosis. Uterus weighed 120 g. No malignancy.

LESSONS

- Learnt clinical and intra-abdominal findings when caesarean site and neighboring area along with bladder gets adherent to the lower abdominal wall.
- Gave clinical material to establish and introduce clinical "cervicofundal" sign and altered sonographic findings to suspect and diagnose the above described specific adhesions.

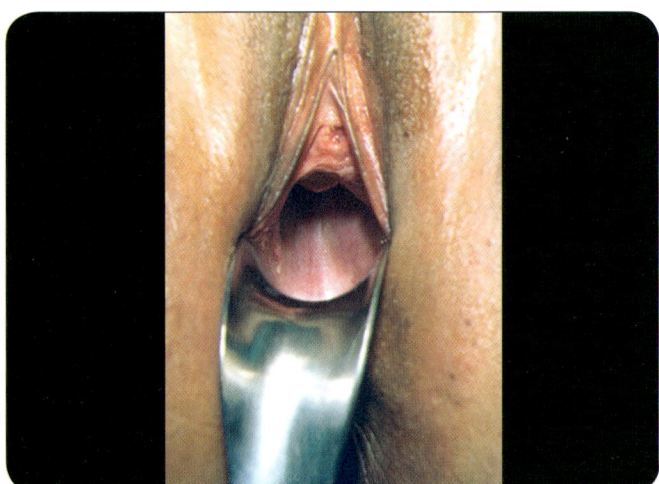

Fig. 1: Speculum examination in a woman with past caesarean sections shows a stretched and pulled up posterior vaginal wall and unseen cervix, high up behind pubic symphysis.[8]

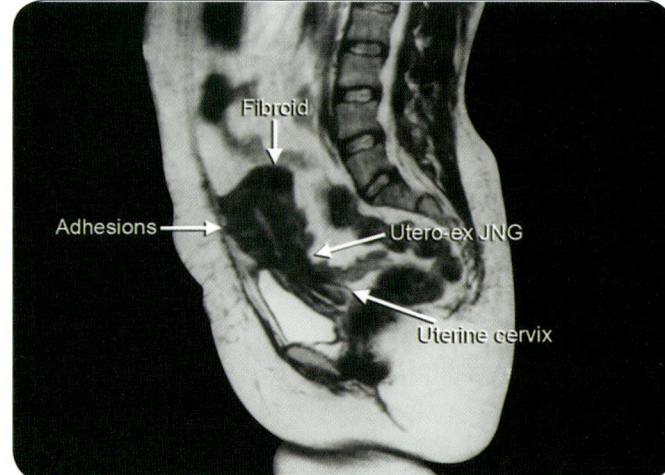

Fig. 2: Magnetic resonance imaging (MRI) shows elongated, displaced cervix behind the symphysis pubis facing the upper third of the vaginal wall and adhesions between the bladder and cervical surfaces.[1]

Section 6: Failed Trial Vaginal Hysterectomy/Trial Vaginal Route

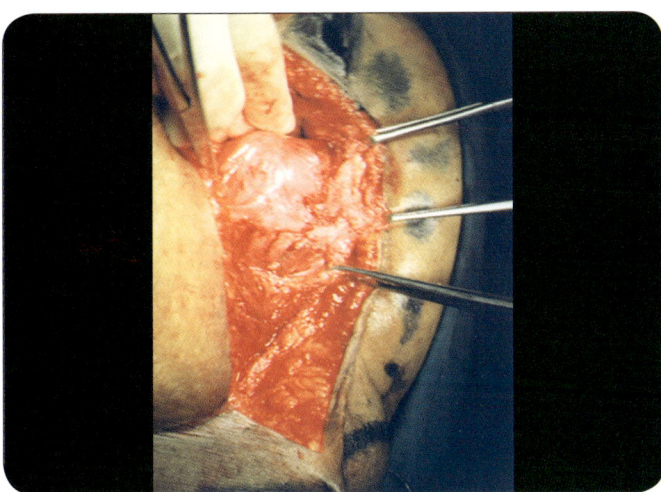

Fig. 3: Classic adhesions following caesarean section seen at laparotomy. Deaver's retractor and Alli's forceps on the skin marking at the umbilical level close to the upper end of the right paramedian incision. The uterine fundus shown by fingers is well above half way between the symphysis pubis and the umbilicus.[8]

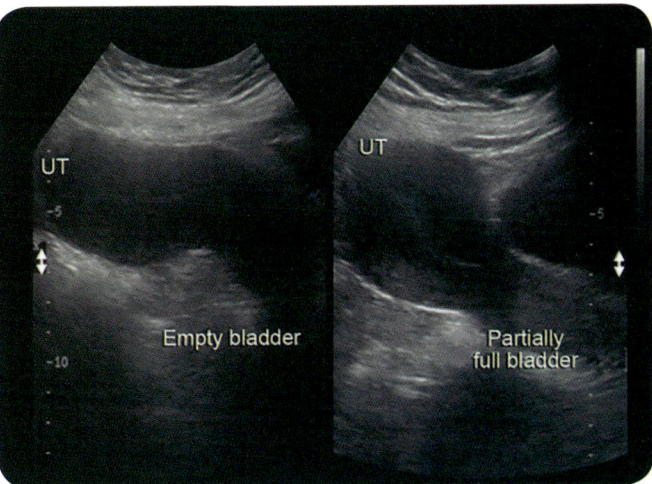

Fig. 4: Transabdominal pelvic sonography with empty bladder and partially full bladder in a patient with prior caesarean section shows effect of elongated cervix.[2]
(UT: Urinary tract).

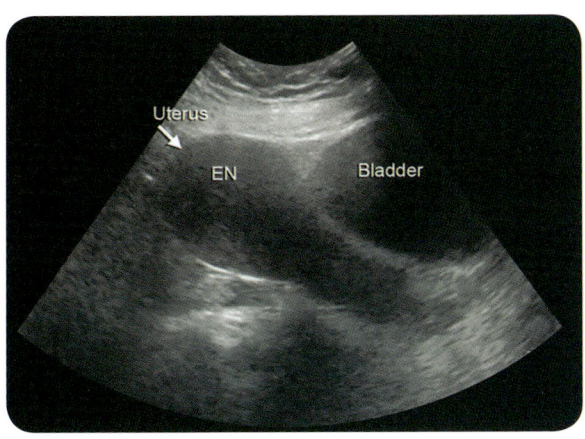

Fig. 5: Transabdominal pelvic sonography with full bladder in a patient with prior caesarean sections. There is absence of a distended urinary bladder between the fundus of the uterus and the anterior lower abdominal wall.[2]

- On speculum examination, cervix was not easily visualized. Cervix remained behind and above sagging the anterior vaginal wall. Posterior vaginal wall was stretched or pulled up. Traction on the cervix "pulled in" the lower abdominal wall or caused dimpling.
- Uterine fundus was disproportionately at a higher level for the uterine size. Opening the abdomen showed lower uterocervical surface and bladder were glued to the lower abdominal wall with obliterated anterior uterocervical pouch and cervix unduly elongated. Sonographically an elongated pulled up cervix, even full bladder does not appear between the fundus of the uterus and anterior abdominal wall and uterus may tend to retroflex.

What inspired: "Trial VH".

LESSON

- Established clinical and later sonographic signs for preoperative diagnosis and as a contraindication for VH.

CASE 56: DIMINISHED "UTERUS-FREE" SPACE (ALTERED UTEROCERVICAL ANGLE)

Name: Mrs. X
Age: 42 years
Parity: 2 FTND (full term normal delivery).
LD: 10 years back

This was a case of an obese, hypertensive and diabetic woman (corpus cancer syndrome) with clinically a 22 weeks size uterus and the fundus just below the umbilicus. A normal cervix like a "butt" with physiological descent of cervix to attempt VH. Fornices were clear.

Sonography: It showed uterine volume of 1,080 cm³ with 16 cm × 12.5 cm × 10 cm dimensions with a large fibroid of 11.5 cm × 11.7 cm × 8 cm and normal adnexae. The patient was taken as "Trial VH" case.[3,4]

Diagnosis: Large uterus with fibroids.

Operation: Failed "Trial VH", abdominal hysterectomy plus prophylactic bilateral salpingectomy (not salpingo-oophorectomy).

What deters/dissuades VH: The large-sized uterus.

Examination under anesthesia revealed the cervix was small like a butt with physiologic descent. The uterus size was 22–24 weeks needing massive debulking. Anteriorly the vesicouterine peritoneum was easily accessed. Pouch of Douglas was distally placed and the posterior peritoneum was accessed at 6″ (inch) from the external os of the cervix. The cervix was bisected to attempt debulking, but that was difficult as too much of lateral vaginal walls retraction was needed. Further cervical descent was zero, the posterior uterine surface was not seen and accessing lateral connections after uterosacrals and Mackendrot's was almost impossible because of the big transverse bulge of the uterus reducing the "uterus free" space. Back flow from blood vessels was an additional disturbing factor. Thus, the "Trial" was given-up and laparotomy performed with low Pfannenstiel's incision. Abdominal hysterectomy was completed without difficulty. The tubes and ovaries appeared normal though both tubes had mild hydrosalpinx. Both ovaries were preserved and bilateral salpingectomy was done. Hemostasis was checked and the abdomen closed. Blood transfusion was not need. Hospital stay was of 5 days and postoperatively there was an uneventful speedy recovery.

At HP, the uterus weighed 1,150 g. Multiple fibroids with severe adenomyosis were seen. Both tubes were normal. No malignancy.

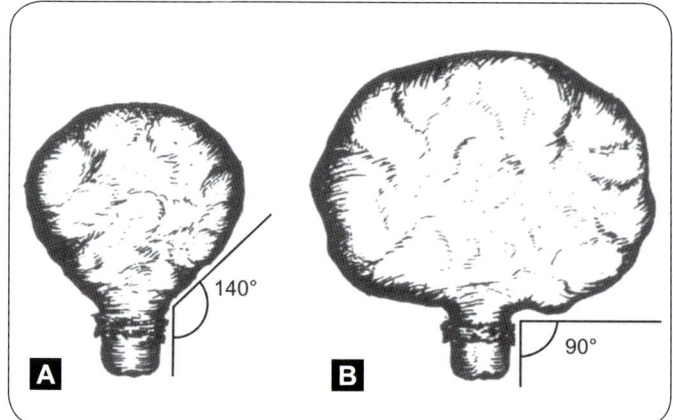

Figs. 1A and B: (A) The depicted angle between the lateral cervical and uterine borders, more than 140°, makes access and reach easier and (B) reduction of the angle towards 90° makes access very difficult or impossible.[9]

Why did "Trial VH" fail? Failure was not only because of the large uterine size but because of position and location of the fibroid that obstructed and reduced the uterus-free space. Because of the large-sized fibroid, in a peculiar position with a disproportionate bulge laterally, posed as an obstruction for the operator to access the uterine vessels and lateral uterine connections for securing them. The bulge continued to cause an obstacle upwards.

The angle between the lateral cervical surface and the ascending uterine wall from the cervix can assist or inhibit surgery. If the angle is obtuse 140° or thereabouts, it facilitates an access to the lateral connections but when the angle gets closer to 90°, chances to get an access to the lateral connections are heavily reduced and failure in VH rises steeply.[4,9,10] Intraoperatively, careful examination by the fingers can prognosticate this. The broader the uterine base above the cervix, the greater the difficulty and chances of failing. In my earlier practice, 4 failures out of 9 were due to altered configuration which made me learn the above and principles to be implemented.[9]

What inspired: Tackle a large-sized uterus.

LESSON

- If all three uterine dimensions are larger than 10–12 cm, it is worth evaluating the site and angle (Figs. 1A and B) of the uterus before considering the case for "Trial VH".

CASE 57: OVARIAN ENDOMETRIOSIS WITH POSITIVE "DIMPLE SIGN"

Name: Mrs. X
Age: 44 years
C/O: Heavy and prolonged menses.
Last menstrual period (LMP): December 2, 2013.

Not obese but with hypertension and diabetes, taking treatment for hypothyroidism.

On clinical examination, uterus was 12+ weeks size. Normal cervix with slightly restricted descent. Left adnexal mass (endometriotic cyst) giving positive Dimple sign[11]—a contraindication to undertake vaginal route for hysterectomy. Right fornix was clear.

Sonography findings: Uterus 11.1 cm × 8.4 cm × 7.4 cm with 8.2 cm × 6.5 cm heterogeneous area in posterior wall, uterine volume 370 cm^3. Left ovary with 2 cm × 2 cm size two cysts with internal echoes—endometriotic cysts. Right ovary was absent with past history of laparoscopic right oophorectomy, appendicectomy followed by laparotomy for colostomy because of rectal trauma. Her CA125 was 427. She was taken as "Trial VH" case.[3,4]

Diagnosis: Uterine adenomyosis with left ovarian endometriosis.

Operation: "Trial VH" → Failed → Abdominal hysterectomy with left salpingo-oophorectomy plus right salpingectomy.

Vaginal hysterectomy started as usual. Anterior peritoneum was accessed easily. Posterior vaginal wall needed extra care and despite a good attempt, posterior uterocervical-broad ligament space could not be safely reached.[6,12] Uterines secured but uterine descent was zero. Lateral connections severed till no further higher access but uterine descent remained zero and uterine body remained upright without showing of posterior uterine wall. Trial was given up as further access was not possible and abdomen was opened with a right paramedian incision (H/O colon surgery). Posterior uterine wall showed adherent bulging adenomyoma 5 cm × 5 cm. Frozen pelvis with bladder badly adherent to the upper uterine surface with fundus adherent to the intestines and omentum posteriorly. Both tubes and left ovary were engulfed in the adhesions. Total abdominal hysterectomy with left salpingo-oophorectomy and right salpingectomy done. For safety, the left ureter was identified and kept away before left salpingo-oophorectomy was done. The general surgeon joined at this stage to see that there was no injury and everything was safe and in order. Hemostasis was checked and abdominal closure done. Blood transfusion was not needed. Hospital stay was 5 days followed by an uneventful recovery.

Histopathology study: It showed uterus with severe adenomyosis weighed 440 g. Left ovarian endometriotic cysts. Both tubes also showed endometriosis. 4 weeks later raised CA125 (427) returned to normal.[13]

What inspired: Successful experience of similar clinical pelvic findings in past.

LESSON

- Dimple sign needs extra respect. If VH is attempted, take it always as "Trial vaginal route" case.

CASE 58: LARGE-SIZED UTERUS

Name: Mrs. X
Age: 43 years
Parity: 2 FTND
C/O: Heavy, painful menses.

Clinically uterus was 24+ weeks size, a healthy cervix with physiological descent of the uterus. Abdominally uterus was mobile, nodular with upper uterine margin a little above the umbilicus. Fornices were clear.
Sonography findings: Normal abdominopelvic findings except for large uterus with multiple fibroids. Uterine dimensions were 15.6 cm × 11.4 cm × 8.5 cm, volume 800 cm³ with left wall fibroid of 8.8 cm × 8.1 cm. Tubes and ovaries were normal.
Diagnosis: Uterine fibroids.
Operation: Trial VH followed by abdominal hysterectomy.[3,4]
What deters or dissuades VH: Large-sized uterus.

Hysterectomy started as usual. Cervix was abnormally elongated and hence uterine vessels were distally placed. After securing them, cervix was bisected to carry out morcellation and enucleation.[14-17] This was continued after bisecting lower uterine walls and securing available lateral connections. Large upper fibroid probably obstructed further surgery. Even though surgery reached close to round ligaments, further access to large fibroid for enucleation was not possible. Considering time taken, almost 90 minutes coupled with inevitable oozing and 10 g Hb%, Trial VH was terminated and it was decided to switch over to the abdominal approach.

Abdominally small Pfannenstiel's incision was taken. It was not difficult to deliver the uterus and complete the hysterectomy as only upper pedicles and residual broad ligament tissues were to be secured. Tubes and ovaries were normal. Prophylactic salpingectomy was performed[18] and both healthy ovaries were preserved. Hemostasis was ensured and after thorough lavage, instruments and mop count the abdomen closed in layers. She was given 1 unit of blood. Postoperative period was uneventful with a speedy recovery. Hospital stay was 4 days.
Histopathology report: It showed uterus weighed 900+ g, multiple fibroids with severe uterine adenomyosis. No malignancy.

Trial VH was attempted based on past experience of having hysterectomized larger uteri. Elongated cervix took away the proximity for the access and large lateral wall fibroid obstructed the higher reach on one side.
What inspired: Trial VH for large-sized uterus.

LESSON

- Elongated cervix and too much bulging of the uterus on one side makes it difficult or well-nigh impossible.

CASE 59: OVARIAN MALIGNANCY

Name: Mrs. X
Age: 64 years
Parity: 1 FTND
LD: 40 years back.
C/O: Lower abdominal pain with loss of appetite.
Not obese with no H/O hypertension or diabetes.
Clinically uterus 6 weeks size, freely mobile. Normal cervix with physiological descent to attempt VH. Right fornix had cystic to firm tender mass encroaching on the posterior fornix. Left and anterior fornices were clear.
Sonography: It showed uterus with 90 cm³ volume. Endometrium 4 mm, right ovarian cyst of 10 cm × 6 cm, multiseptation including thick septum but without solid area. Resistance index was 0.6. Left tube and ovary normal. CA125 was normal (30).
Diagnosis: Right ovarian tumor.
Operation: VH with bilateral salpingo-oophorectomy → Right ovarian adenocarcinoma → Failed 'Trial vaginal route' → Abdominal omentectomy and lymph nodes removal, etc.

This was discussed at length, including frozen HP, during vaginal surgery. Well-informed consent was taken and the patient was taken as 'Trial vaginal route' case.[3,4] Patient was keen not to have abdomen opened and without definitive finding to indicate malignancy. VH was straightforward. After uterines were secured, on reaching both upper pedicles, all lateral connections on left were cut to make the uterus free on the left side. Left tube and ovary were normal. Plastic sheet was spread all over the operative field to spare contamination. Right ovarian surface was without excrescences and adhesions. Suprapubic pressure aided by uterine traction exteriorized the right ovarian mass. Thus, hysterectomy was completed along with right salpingo-oophorectomy including intact ovarian mass. Cut open uterus showed normal endometrium. Uterus with right tube and ovary sent for frozen HP study to find out ovarian pathology. The frozen section analysis should be done by an experienced pathologist and the possible predictive factors affecting a false diagnosis should carefully be taken into consideration.[19] Meanwhile contralateral left salpingo-oophorectomy was completed.[8,20-21] Frozen HP reported ovarian malignancy, well-differentiated adenocarcinoma. Matter was discussed and explained to husband and relatives. After collecting peritoneal and lavage fluid for cystological study, vaginal closure was done and she was put in position for laparotomy. Abdomen was opened by a right paramedian incision. Necessary inspection showed normal findings. Required omentectomy with bilateral pelvic lymphadenectomy was done. Liver, diaphragm, para-aortic and inferior vena caval areas were normal. Fluid from para-colic gutters and peritoneal cavity was collected for cytology and closure done. She had an uneventful postoperative recovery.

Paraffin HP reported a well-differentiated adenocarcinoma of right ovary with normal tubes, left ovary and uterus. Uterus weighed 110 g and showed no abnormality. Lymph nodes and omentum were negative for malignancy.

She was referred to an oncosurgeon for opinion before subjecting her to chemotherapy. While dealing with adnexal pathology, particularly ovarian, it is essential to have extra bit of preoperative counseling, informed consent and keep availability of frozen HP study and laparotomy to spare from an untoward aftermath.

What inspired: Absence of solid area on sonography and normal CA125 with facility for frozen HP study.

LESSONS

- Frozen HP and readiness to switch over to laparotomy is mandatory, when ovarian mass is not definitively benign. One learns from mistakes.
- Taking her as 'TRIAL vaginal route' was less disturbing.

REFERENCES

1. Sheth SS, Goyal MV, Shah N. Uterocervical displacement following adhesions after caesarean section. J Gynecol Surg. 1997;13:143-7.
2. Sheth SS, Shah NM, Varaiya D. A sonographic and clinical sign to detect specific adhesions following caesarean section. J Gynecol Surg. 2008;24:27-35.
3. Sheth SS. Vaginal hysterectomy. In: Studd J (Ed). Progress in Obstetrics and Gynecology, 10th edition. London, UK: Churchill Livingstone; 1993. pp. 317-40.
4. Sheth SS, Paghdiwalla KP, Hajari AR. Vaginal route: a gynaecological route for much more than hysterectomy. Best Pract Res Clin Obstet Gynaecol. 2011;25(2):115-32.
5. Sheth SS, Malpani AN. Vaginal hysterectomy following previous caesarean section. Int J Gynecol Obstet. 1995;50:165-9.
6. Sheth SS. Access to vesicouterine and rectouterine pouches. In: Sheth SS (Ed). Vaginal Hysterectomy, 2nd edition. New Delhi, India: Jaypee Brothers Medical Publishers (P) Ltd; 2014. pp. 31-50.

7. Sheth SS. Observations from a FIGO Past President on vaginal hysterectomy and related surgery by the vaginal route. Int J Gynecol Obstet. 2016;135:1-4.
8. Sheth SS. Vaginal hysterectomy. 2005;19(3):307-32.
9. Sheth SS. Uterine fibroids. In: Sheth SS, Studd JW (Eds). Vaginal Hysterectomy. London, UK: Martin Dunitz Ltd; 2002. pp. 79-94.
10. Sheth SS, Rathi MR. Uterine fibroids. In: Sheth SS (Ed). Vaginal Hysterectomy, 2nd edition. New Delhi, India: Jaypee Brothers Medical Publishers (P) Ltd; 2014. pp. 72-89.
11. Sheth SS. Vaginal dimple--a sign of ovarian endometriosis. J Obstet Gynecol. 1991;11;292.
12. Sheth SS. A surgical window to access the obliterated posterior cul-de-sac at vaginal hysterectomy. Int J Gynecol Obstet. 2009;107:244-7.
13. Sheth SS, Ray SS. Severe adenomyosis and CA125. J Obstet Gynecol. 2014;34:79-81.
14. Pelosi MA III, Pelosi MA. The Pryor technique of uterine morcellation. Int J Gynecol Obstet. 1997;58:299-303.
15. Pelosi MA, Pelosi MA III. A comprehensive approach to morcellation of the large uterus. Contemp Obstet Gynecol. 1997;42:106-25.
16. Pelosi MA II, Pelosi MA III. Uterine debulking at vaginal hysterectomy. In: Sheth SS (Ed). Vaginal Hysterectomy, 2nd edition. New Delhi, India: Jaypee Brothers Medical Publishers (P) Ltd; 2014. pp. 90-109.
17. Sheth SS. Rathi MR. Uterine fibroids. In: Sheth SS (Ed). aginal Hysterectomy, 2nd edition. New Delhi, India: Jaypee Brothers Medical Publishers (P) Ltd; 2014. pp. 72-89.
18. Kwon JS, Tinker A, Pansegrau G, McAlpine J, Housty M, McCullum M, et al. Prophylactic salpingectomy and delayed oophorectomy as an alternative for BRCA mutation carriers. Obstet Gynecol. 2013;121(1):14-24.
19. Gultekin E, Gultekin OE, Cingilioglu B, Sayhan S, Sanci M, Yildirim Y. The value of frozen section evaluation in the management of borderline ovarian tumors. J Cancer Res Ther. 2011;7(4):416-20.
20. Sheth SS. Adnexectomy for benign pathology at vaginal hysterectomy without laparoscopic assistance. Br J Obstet Gynecol. 2002;109:1401-5.
21. Sheth SS. Adnexal pathology at vaginal hysterectomy? In: Sheth SS (Ed). Vaginal Hysterectomy, 2nd edition. New Delhi, India: Jaypee Brothers Medical Publishers (P) Ltd; 2014. pp. 150-62.

CASE 60: UTERINE BULK IMPEDES DESCENT

Name: Mrs. BA
Age: 40 years
Parity: FT (full term) SVD (spontaneous vaginal delivery) × 1
Indications for surgery: Mass effect, menorrhagia and anemia.
Medical/surgical comorbidity: Chronic hypertension.
Operative time: 4 hours (inclusive of cystoscopy and uterosacral colposuspension).
Hemoglobin (Hb) pre- and postoperative: 10.7 g/dL, 6.8 g/dL.
Recovery course: 2 units packed red blood cell (PRBC) transfused, day 2 discharge with Hb 9.1 g/dL.
Pathology report: Benign oviducts, uterus 2,214 g, leiomyoma [add 10% to uterine weight, specimen sent directly in formalin to pathology. Gross weight directly in operation room (OR) would be 10–15% more].
Preoperative evaluation: Mobile uterus all directions, readily accessed cervix, roomy pelvis, benign endometrial biopsy. Magnetic resonance imaging (MRI) showed anterior myoma 6 cm with distal margin just apical to internal os anteriorly, a 10 cm posterior myoma with distal margin 3 cm apical to cervix, two large fundal myomas 10 cm each, and diffuse multiple small myomas.

Patient appropriately counseled for "Trial vaginal hysterectomy (VH)" with high likelihood of ultimate abdominal operation.
What deters/dissuades: Uterine bulk.
Surgery: Sharp entry posterior into Douglas and anterior below bladder into vesicouterine space (VUS), followed by division of uterosacral and cardinal pedicles was easily accomplished. This was to be expected given preoperative assessment of cervix and vagina, and the absence of risk factors for adhesions. Plan at this point was to progress apical to the 6 cm myoma, inject with vasopressin and enucleate, then secure the uterine artery pedicles and attempt to morcellate from there. However, this plan did not materialize as the anterior lower segment myoma was just out of reach apically and behind pubis. Cervix was amputated and vaginal cuff was closed. A 10 cm Maylard incision on the abdomen was made (rectus muscle attachments to its fascial sheath and linea alba are fully preserved while the muscle is transversely divided with cautery). Vasopressin was injected intramyometrial, and fibroid enucleation and morcellation proceeded rapidly until uterus was delivered. Lateral pedicles of utero-ovarian, round, and uterine artery were all clamped and cut. After the specimen was removed the clamped pedicles were sutured, the pelvis irrigated, and abdomen closed.

LESSONS

- Starting the surgery vaginally facilitated an easier, faster, safer and more cosmetic abdominal operation. Total abdominal hysterectomy (TAH) with a uterus this size would have involved a very large transverse, or even vertical incision. Instead, the most challenging parts of the abdominal operation involving the deep pelvis were addressed at the surgery outset by starting the case vaginally. The bladder was separated off from the lower uterine segment, the deep pelvic pedicles were divided, and the vaginal cuff closed. The abdominal incision could thus be smaller, since access into deep pelvis was no longer required. Cardinal ligament division vaginally, laterally displaces the ureters from the uterine arteries, thereby near eliminating all risk for ureter injury during abdominal approach to the uterine pedicles.
- Patient counseling is critical and the surgeon going into the operating theater with a sound plan of attack are essential with "Trial VH". One must also remember that a "Failed Trial" is not failure. In the end, this patient was quite satisfied. She was given a small opportunity as opposed to no opportunity for a minimal invasive surgery, and the invasive procedure she ultimately got was less invasive and anatomically safer that had TAH been pursued at outset.

CASE 61: EXTENSIVE ADHESIONS FROM PID (PELVIC INFLAMMATORY DISEASE) LIMITS DESCENT FOR VH

Name: Mrs. LO
Age: 41 years
Parity: FT SVD × 1
Indication for surgery: Mass effect, menorrhagia and severe anemia.
Medical/surgical comorbidity: Body mass index (BMI) 46, chronic hypertension.
Operative time: 4 hours 20 minutes
Hb pre- and postoperative: 8.1 g/dL, 8.3 g/dL (2 units transfused intraoperatively)
Recovery course: Discharge day 3
Pathology report: Acute and chronic salpingitis, uterus 727 g, leiomyoma (add 10% to uterine weight, specimen sent directly in formalin to pathology. Gross weight directly in OR would be 10–15% more).
Preoperative evaluation: Patient admitted to hospital 1 month prior to surgery with Hb 4 g/dL. Reported long-standing above symptoms. She was transfused and underwent examination under anesthesia followed by hysteroscopy and endometrial sampling. A mobile 20 week uterus with dominant bulk posterior and readily accessible cervix was noted.
What deters/dissuades: Uterine bulk.
Surgery: Anterior VUS entry was easily accomplished. Posterior entry was unsuccessful. Dissection proceeded apically and division of uterosacral, cardinal and uterine artery pedicles were all accomplished extraperitoneal. Neither cul-de-sac peritoneum was able to be entered. Eventually a small posterior peritoneal window expressed chocolate fluid and deep rectal palpation confirmed an obliterated cul-de-sac. Although neither culd-des-sac had been entered, uterine descent was deemed sufficient to bivalve the cervix up into the lower segment and begin an intrauterine morcellation. However, exposure was too limited to access the most distal large myoma, and when some moderate bleeding was encountered the vaginal approach was abandoned.

The cervix was amputated and a sponge packing was placed apical to vaginal cuff, achieving hemostasis. Uterosacral colposuspension, cystoscopy and vaginal cuff closure were performed before converting abdominally.

A transverse 7 cm Maylard abdominal incision was performed, with recti divided only 3 cm on each side, leaving intact both epigastric vessels and attachments of recti to fascia and linea alba. Omental adhesions to uterus and bilateral adnexa were divided. The right adnexa was densely adherent to pelvic sidewall and left adnexa was sucked down in adhesions deep in the pelvis. There were bowel and omental adhesions posteriorly to the uterus that were divided sharply. The uterus was then incised and a large myoma removed. Morcellation was relatively bloodless as the uterine pedicles had already been vaginally secured. With uterine decompression delivery through the abdominal incision was achieved. This faciliated exposure and sharp division of remaining intraperitoneal uterine adhesions. At this point, all lateral pedicles of utero-ovarian, round and broad ligament were able to be divided and uterus was removed. Exposure was now sufficient to locate and remove the packing that was inserted vaginally and then address the adnexal adhesiolysis. The right adnexa was freed from the sidewall and the left from the floor of the deep pelvis. Both oviducts were very abnormally dilated and tortuous, and bilateral salpingectomy was performed.

LESSONS

- Nothing in the patient's history suggested this level of adhesive disease. Pelvic examination in an obese patient can be somewhat limited. That the uterus remained mobile on examination is likely due to its large mass, and that no serosal adhesions directly to pelvic sidewall or abdominal wall were present.
- Note again how initiating the case vaginally, completing all the necessary work in deep pelvis to begin the operation, facilitates a much easier, safer, cosmetic, and hemostatic abdominal operation should that be necessary.

CASE 62: UNANTICIPATED UTERINE ADHESIONS TO ABDOMINAL WALL-1

Name: Mrs. YS
Age: 48 years
Parity: FT SVD × 1, FT caesarean × 1
Indication for surgery: Dysmenorrhea, menorrhagia and anemia.
Medical/surgical comorbidity: BMI 43, asthma and chronic hypertension.
Operative time: 2 hours 20 minutes (inclusive of cystoscopy and uterosacral colposuspension).
Hb pre- and postoperative: 10.8 g/dL, 9 g/dL
Recovery course: Discharged day 1, rapid recovery.
Pathology report: Fallopian tubes with endometriosis, uterus 185 g, adenomyosis and leiomyoma (add 10% to uterine weight, specimen sent directly in formalin to pathology. Gross weight directly in OR would be 10–15% more).
Preoperative evaluation: Patient presented requesting hysterectomy after having failed treatment elsewhere with nonsurgical options. She had a recent benign endometrial biopsy.

Cervix was readily accessible and uterus palpated 8–10 weeks size with mobility, but examination somewhat limited by habitus. Patient appropriately counseled regarding "Trial VH".
What deters/dissuades: Prior caesarean.
Surgery: Accessing *broad ligament space* bilaterally allowed for safe anterior entry to VUS and division of caesarean scar. Posterior entry was easily accomplished. Lateral pedicle division proceeded accordingly and uterine arteries were secured. Cervix was noted to be markedly elongated, raising concern for abdominal wall adhesions. The left adnexa pedicle was identified and divided vaginally but no further uterine descent followed. The right adnexa could not be visualized or manually identified prompting decision to abort.

The cervix was amputated, uterosacral colposuspension performed followed by cystoscopy, and the vaginal cuff closed. Abdominally, a 5 cm transverse minilaparotomy with transverse rectus muscle division was performed. The peritoneum was entered from a most lateral position to avoid central adhesions. Adhesions of omentum to abdominal wall were divided to gain exposure, at which point very dense fundal-abdominal wall adhesions were lysed. The right upper pedicles were divided and uterus removed. The ovaries were inspected and bilateral salpingectomy performed.

LESSONS

- An elongated cervix encountered at surgery in a patient without advanced uterine prolapse is a red flag for dense abdominal wall adhesions.
- Preoperative pelvic examinations are not always reliable in obese patients.
- Number of caesareans does not necessarily correlate with extent of adhesions, and if adhesions are present, a small uterus, because it is smaller, is more likely to have those adhesions extend to fundus. A uterus with dense fundus-abdominal wall adhesions is usually impossible to deliver vaginally.
- Obese patients derive the most benefit from a vaginal operation, because they are hard to position laparoscopically, and their complication risk from abdominal surgery is so high. By starting vaginally, even though uterus could not be delivered, it facilitated a minilaparotomy and a recovery course postoperative more in line with minimal invasive surgery.

CASE 63: UNANTICIPATED UTERINE ADHESIONS TO ABDOMINAL WALL-2

Name: Mrs. EM
Age: 48 years
Parity: 1 FT caesarean
Indication for surgery: Menorrhagia, dysmenorrhea and chronic pelvic pain.
Medical/surgical comorbidity: BMI 35
Operative time: 4 hours 20 minutes (inclusive of cystoscopy and uterosacral colposuspension).
Hb pre- and postoperative: 12.8 g/dL, 10.3 g/dL
Recovery course: Day 2 hospital discharge. Home convalescence for 3 weeks before return to full activity.
Pathology report: Bilateral oviducts with chronic inflammation, uterus 140 g, leiomyoma (add 10% to uterine weight, specimen sent directly in formalin to pathology. Gross weight directly in OR would be 10–15% more).
Preoperative evaluation: Chronic symptoms as noted above, desirous of definitive management with hysterectomy. Counseled for "Trial VH". Examination findings are limited by habitus but revealed a readily accessed cervix and 10-week size uterus.
What deters/dissuades: Prior caesarean.
Surgery: Posterior entry unsuccessful initially, and peritoneum noted to be somewhat indurated. Entry bilateral into *broad ligament space* facilitated central scar division of bladder and access into VUS. Extraperitoneal division of all lower pedicles and uterine arteries was performed. At this point, entry was achieved through posterior peritoneum. The uterus however was very resistant to further descent, and the cervix appeared somewhat elongated (~5 cm). The problem of resistance was anterior behind pubis and patient had no history of uterine myoma. Cervix was amputated to allow better visualization of lower segment and fundus, but immediately upon doing so the uterus rapidly retracted from view and attempts to visualize it again were futile.

Uterosacral colposuspension, cystoscopy, and vaginal cuff closure was performed.

An 8 cm transverse abdominal incision was made through the old caesarean scar. The rectus sheath was transversely opened and rectus muscles were divided with cautery transversely for half their width, thus sparing the epigastric vessels. The peritoneum was opened transversely from a lateral position to avoid central adhesions. Extensive adhesiolysis was required to free the uterus from abdominal wall, and bladder from uterus. There were also significant adnexal adhesions suggestive of previous pelvic inflammatory disease. After completing all adhesiolysis the upper lateral pedicles were divided and uterus delivered. The ovaries were evaluated and a bilateral salpingectomy performed.

LESSONS

- These extensive adhesions were unexpected. It is important to familiarize oneself with "Sheth Cervicofundal sign". However, extensive adhesions do not necessarily present themselves in an obvious way preoperatively, and especially so when dealing with the limitations present when examining obese patients.
- This case could and should have been converted abdominally sooner. There is no reason to struggle heroically for a vaginal delivery once dense abdominal wall adhesions are suggested by the anatomy. Signs to look for are anterior resistance to descent and an elongated cervix (in a patient without a pre-existing advanced prolapse).

CASE 64: UNANTICIPATED UTERINE ADHESIONS TO ABDOMINAL WALL-3

Name: Mrs. ED
Age: 43 years
Parity: 1 FT caesarean
Indication for surgery: Chronic pelvic pain and menorrhagia.
Medical/surgical comorbidity: BMI 31
Operative time: 4 hours (inclusive of cystoscopy and uterosacral colposuspension).
Hb pre- and postoperative: 11.4 g/dL, 7.5 g/dL
Recovery course: Day 3 discharge, and 2-week home convalescence before full return to activity.
Pathology report: Benign oviducts, uterus 153 g, leiomyoma (add 10% to uterine weight, specimen sent directly in formalin to pathology. Gross weight directly in OR would be 10–15% more).
Preoperative evaluation: Patient presented desirous of definitive surgical management for her long-standing complaints as noted. Benign endometrial biopsy obtained. Cervix readily accessed, uterus 10-week size, seemingly mobile.

Counseled and consented for "Trial VH".
What deters/dissuades: Prior caesarean.
Surgery: Easy posterior entry. Anterior VUS entry was facilitated by dissection into *broad ligament space* and sharp dissection through caesarean scar between bladder and lower segment uterus. Anterior dissection was reevaluated and advanced apically below bladder following each pedicle division. After dividing and securing the cardinal ligaments, it was noted that there was very minimal descent of the uterine body. Only the cervix was descending, and it appeared elongated, which was not consistent with patient's history and raised concern for fundal abdominal wall adhesions.

However, further progress was attempted. The uterine arteries were reached, divided and secured. The cervix was bivalved, the myometrium wedge resected and the dominant myoma removed. But despite these efforts, the added descent obtained was ultimately insufficient to access the dissection plane between fundus and abdominal wall. After amputating cervix, performing colposuspension followed by cystoscopy and then completing closure of vaginal cuff, the surgery was moved abdominally.

A 6 cm transverse incision through the patient's old transverse lower abdominal scar was made and dense subcutaneous scarring was encountered and divided. In Maylard fashion, the rectus sheath was transversely divided and, without undermining fascia attachment to rectus muscles, division of the muscles proceeded accordingly with cautery for transverse length of the incision, and the peritoneum entered from lateral perspective to avoid central adhesions. These adhesions were extremely dense involving uterus, right adnexa, abdominal wall and part of bladder dome. Careful sharp dissection through this scar freed uterus from abdominal wall, thus allowing for pedicle division and specimen delivery. However, the process of trying to free the scar partially deserosalized bladder dome (which was then repaired by the surgeon with interrupted chromic) and compromised the right infundibulopelvic (IP) ligament (requiring sacrifice of the right ovary). The left adnexa was separately located encased in dense scar in the deep pelvis. This was freed up with sharp dissection, allowing for inspection of that ovary and left salpingectomy.

LESSON

- See above Cases 62 and 63.

CASE 65: PARASITIC MYOMA AND INACCESSIBLE ADNEXA LEADS TO LAPAROSCOPIC COMPLETION OF VH

Name: Mrs. KC
Age: 37 years
Parity: 0
Indication for surgery: Mass effect and menorrhagia.
Medical/surgical comorbidity: BMI 31
Operative time: 3 hours 40 minutes (inclusive of cystoscopy and uterosacral colposuspension).
Hb pre- and postoperative: 12.9 g/dL, 8.4 g/dL
Recovery course: Day 1 discharge, analgesics × 1 week, rapid return to baseline activity.
Pathology report: Benign oviducts, uterus 290 g, fibroids (add 10% to uterine weight, specimen sent directly in formalin to pathology. Gross weight directly in OR would be 10–15% more).
Preoperative course: Patient expressed that she had no interest in fertility and desired for definitive management with hysterectomy to resolve her long-standing reported symptoms. A benign endometrial biopsy was obtained prior to surgery.
What deters/dissuades: Nulliparity together with enlarged uterus.
Surgery: Cervicouterine junction was very narrow, while fundal myomas were quite broad. There was difficulty gaining descent for morcellation, and there was bleeding encountered from vessels directly feeding the myomas. Despite this steady bleeding, the decision was made to pursue morcellation once it was confirmed that the main uterine vessel branches were secured. The cervix was bivaled up to the lower segment and the dominant myoma identified with large anterior retropubic component. Wedge resection of this anterior myoma was continued until the entire tumor was pulled under pubic bone and delivered—along with the remaining uterine tissue. Clamping of the upper pedicles finally achieved hemostasis. However, neither adnexa was readily visible and a fibroid 3 cm diameter on patient's right appeared adherent to pelvic sidewall and not readily accessible for vaginal removal. The vaginal cuff was closed and the surgery converted to laparoscopy. Adnexae at laparoscopy were found to be grossly normal but pulled superiorly out of pelvis. The myoma noted earlier was adherent to pelvic sidewall with a parasitic blood supply from IP ligament. Laparoscopic bilateral salpingectomy and myomectomy was performed, concluding the operation.

LESSONS

- Multiple factors come into play when assessing surgical challenges. This case involved a uterus under 300 g, but the patient was nulliparous and descent was limited, the uterus had mostly anterior bulk and a "cannonball" fundal contour coming off a stalk-like junction of cervix with lower uterine segment. Delivering this uterus vaginally was more difficult than other listed cases involving uteri more than twice as large.
- This case also nicely represents "the exception that proves the rule" that younger patients without adhesive disease have readily accessible adnexa via vaginal route.
- Here we have a young patient without adhesions with inaccessible adnexa. This in turn led to inaccessibility of the myoma parasitically fed by the IP ligament, warranting unexpected laparoscopic conversion at case end.
- Another general rule is that morcellation can proceed relatively bloodless following division of uterine arteries. Here we have a case post-uterine artery division where accessory vasculature coming from the adnexa and directly feeding a fundal myomas led to a morcellation process that was fairly bloody.

Section 7
SPECIAL CASES: VAGINAL HYSTERECTOMY

"Men often become what they believe themselves to be. If I believe I cannot do something, it makes me incapable of doing it. But when I believe I can, then I acquire the ability to do it even if I didn't have it in the beginning".
— Mahatma Gandhi

CASES

Dr Shirish S Sheth

Case 66: VH Plus H/O Rupture Uterus and Two Caesarean Sections
Case 67: VH Plus Broad Ligament Myomectomy without Laparoscopy Plus Contralateral Endometriotic Cyst
Case 68: VH for CIN III
Case 69: VH for Metastatic Breast Cancer Plus Uterine Adenomyosis
Case 70: VH: Prophylactic for Hydatidiform Mole
Case 71: VH with BSO for Twisted Ovarian Cyst
Case 72: VH for Uterine Fibroids with H/O Failed Abdominal Hysterectomy
Case 73: VH under Local Anesthesia for Pulmonary Fibrosis
Case 74: VH with Altered Approach to VUP (VH with BSO)
Case 75: VH with Bicornuate Uterus
Case 76: Bladder Stone Removal at VH Plus Anterior and Posterior Repair

Dr Seth Finkelstein

Case 77: Vaginal Hysterectomy as Emergency Procedure for Cornual Ectopic Pregnancy
Case 78: Vaginal Supracervical Hysterectomy 10 Years after Mesh Hysteropexy

Dr Carl W Zimmerman

Case 79: Vaginal Hysterectomy (VH): Incarcerated Prolapse due to Cervical Leiomyoma and an Intramural Myoma
Case 80: VH in Nullipara with Ongoing Chemotherapy for Non-gynecologic Malignancies
Case 81: VH for Endometrial Carcinoma in Morbidly Obese with History of Caesarean Section

CASE 66: VH PLUS H/O RUPTURE UTERUS AND TWO CAESAREAN SECTIONS

Name: Mrs. X
Age: 41 years
Parity: 4 (1st FTCS, 2nd rupture uterus and 3rd and 4th Elective caesarean sections).

She had her first confinement by caesarean section followed by a ruptured uterus in the lower uterine segment during her second pregnancy for which the uterus was sutured and preserved wihtout tubal sterilization. Following the rupture in the uterus in the past, she had two elective caesarean sections for her next two pregnancies.[1,2]

She now had 8-week size uterus with menorrhagia not responding to medical treatment and three dilation and curettages (D&Cs) had been done which showed a benign endometrium. In between, the hemoglobin had fallen to 6.5 g. She was keen to have her uterus removed and she did not want to have her abdomen cut again.

Earlier, it was explained to her that she could have a long-acting intrauterine device (IUD) or endometrial ablation to avoid surgery. She was even offered laparoscopic bilateral oophorectomy but she declined that as well as opening of the abdomen for hysterectomy. She requested and pleaded for hysterectomy via the vaginal route to spare her abdomen. In fact, she said that she had travelled to Mumbai (Bombay) from a small place in Gujarat State to avoid abdominal surgery. This was the inspiration to attempt a hysterectomy via the vaginal route in such a rare case and to establish the credibility of the route and technique.

Clinically, there was a freely mobile 8-week size uterus without pelvic pathology, i.e. labeled as dysfunctional uterine bleeding (DUB) of the past. Sonography showed a uterine volume of 130 cm^3, adenomyotic with other normal findings. The same was confirmed under anesthesia and a decision taken to go for hysterectomy by the vaginal route.

I asked myself, in absence of the previously ruptured uterus and caesarean sections and based on the findings obtained at clinical examination and examination under anesthesia, would I have attempted vaginal hysterectomy (VH)? If the answer was yes, then one can attempt a hysterectomy via the vaginal route as a "Trial VH" case.[3-5]

However, this being rare and unreported earlier in the literature,[6] in case any complication occurred because of the VH, the blame and universal comment would be "Why was laparoscopic or abdominal hysterectomy not done?" Therefore, evaluatory or diagnostic laparoscopy was performed to get a crystal clear picture of the interior and to avoid complication. Laparoscopic evaluation found nothing contraindicating the vaginal route and boosted confidence to undertake VH.

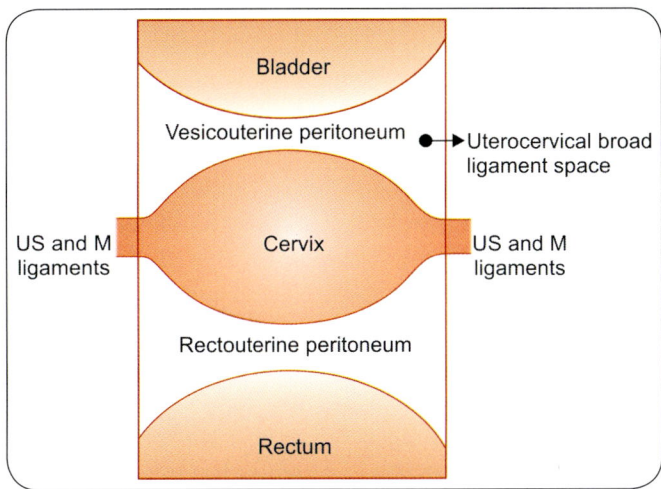

Fig. 1: This figure distinctly shows the space between bladder and cervix or cervicouterine surface, which is much more under lateral one-fifth of bladder when compared with central three-fifths of bladder.[4]

Diagnosis: Abnormal uterine bleeding with past history of (H/O) rupture uterus and caesarean sections.
Operation: VH with bilateral salpingo-oophorectomy (BSO).
What deters or dissuades: H/O rupture of uterus in the past.

Vaginal hysterectomy was performed without difficulty. Because of three caesarean sections and the ruptured uterus on one occasion, the vesicouterine peritoneum (VUP) or the bladder separation was achieved via the uterocervical-broad ligament space (Fig. 1)[5-11] and hysterectomy completed as per routine. Advantageously access to VUP was easy. The patient was very keen to have her ovaries removed and hopefully have no more surgeries in life, particularly of the genital tract. Therefore, concomitant BSO was performed at her request. Hemostasis was checked and vaginal closure done.

Blood loss was less than 50 mL. She had an uneventful speedy recovery from the surgery and went home in Mumbai after 1 day. Postoperative follow-up showed excellent results.

Histopathology (HP): It showed a uterus that weighed 160 g with severe adenomyosis, with normal tubes and ovaries. No malignancy.

It is worth keeping in mind that 80% of the world do not have a laparoscope and/or laparoscopist and a woman may refuse any more opening of the abdomen.[12] Fortunately rupture of uterus is so rare in the affluent world and consideration of vaginal route for hysterectomy for such past history is rarer.

Kovac et al.[13] suggest laparoscopically-assisted VH (LAVH) for gaining entry through a scarred anterior culde-sac after caesarean section. Coulum and Pratt[14] believe that the chief concern centers on bladder injury and difficulty in gaining entry through the scarred anterior culde-sac. The adhesions between the bladder and the lower uterine segment, particularly after caesarean section in the past can be dense or tough in the midline but not laterally.[4,7] Let an H/O caesarean section in the past be not taken as an excuse to avoid VH. Entry from the free-lateral space, i.e. uterocervical-broad ligament space can easily pave the way. However, adhesions following ruptured uterus is unknown or anyone's guess. Therefore, diagnostic laparoscopy was performed.

What inspired:
- The patient's desperate plea to keep the abdomen intact
- With same clinical findings in the absence of past H/O caesarean sections and rupture uterus, I would have taken her for VH.

LESSONS

- Zeal to meet the rare challenge
- At least, to never take H/O caesarean section as a contraindication or get dissuaded by it.

CASE 67: VH PLUS BROAD LIGAMENT MYOMECTOMY WITHOUT LAPAROSCOPY PLUS CONTRALATERAL ENDOMETRIOTIC CYST

Name: Mrs. X
Age: 51 years
Parity: 2 FTND (full term normal delivery)
Last delivery (LD): 20 years back
Complains of (C/O): Heavy and painful menses

Clinically uterus 14-week size, mobile and nodular, normal cervix with physiological descent to attempt VH. Right ovarian cyst and left adnexal firm mass.

Sonography: It revealed uterus with volume of 270 cm^3 with right ovarian endometriotic cyst of 3.9 cm × 3.7 cm × 2.9 cm plus left broad ligament fibroid 4.5 cm × 2.8 cm. Left ovary normal.

Diagnosis: Uterine adenomyosis with right ovarian endometrial cyst plus left broad ligament fibroid.[15]

Operation: VH, BSO and broad ligament myomectomy without laparoscopy.

What deters/dissuades: Broad ligament fibroid.

Access to VUP was easy. Access to the pouch of Douglas (POD) or posterior pouch needed extra careful surgery. It was distorted by ovarian endometriosis and needed a good attempt to get a plane of cleavage. It was accessed by attempting to reach posterior cervico broad ligament space after getting posterior cervicouterine surface free of soft tissue and felt firm cervix directly.[4,16] Uterine debulking and all-round necessary adhesiolysis was done and both the tubes and ovaries were freed for BSO.[17] As per routine, uterus was freed on the normal left adnexal side by cutting all the lateral connections—left upper pedicle.

Traction on the free uterus on one side facilitated salpingo-oophorectomy of the right pathological adnexa. On naked eye examination, cut open uterus was normal except for its size. This was followed by salpingo-oophorectomy of the contralateral normal left adnexa and completed the hysterectomy with BSO. This brought the broad ligament fibroid on the left closer for the operator. Left broad ligament fibroid was easily felt and seen bulging. Anatomy was respected and the capsule of the fibroid was very carefully cut to enucleate the fibroid. Small bleeders were cauterized to have hemostasis. Access and enucleation of broad ligament fibroid were straightforward.[15,18-21] Hemostasis was checked and vaginal closure done. Blood transfusion was not needed. Hospital stay was 2 days with speedy postoperative recovery.

Histopatholgy: It showed uterus weighed 290 g, severely adenomyotic. Right endometriotic cyst. Left ovary and both tubes were normal. Left broad ligament fibroid weighed 46 g. No malignancy.

What inspired: Experience of salpingo-oophorectomy at VH.

LESSONS

- Broad ligament myomectomy at VH was easier than concomitant salpingo-oophorectomy at VH. Spared the abdomen and laparoscope.
- Broad ligament myomectomy added flavor.

CASE 68: VH FOR CIN III

Name: Mrs. X
Age: 43 years
Parity: 3 FTND
LD: 18 years back
C/O: Spotting and blood-stained discharge per vaginam. Clinically 6-week size uterus. Cervix with erosion on both lips, spotting easily on touch but there was no ulcer or growth. Favorable cervical descent to attempt VH. Fornices were clear.
Sonography: It showed slightly enlarged uterus, 110 cm^3 volume with normal adnexal area.

"Pap" smear showed transformation zone with several cells showing mildly enlarged and pleomorphic atypical nuclei. Cervical biopsies showed high-grade cervical intraepithelial neoplasia (CIN) III without invasion or invasive cancer. Biopsy slides were rechecked by senior reliable histopathologist to confirm the same. This was explained at length to the patient and her husband. She intended taking no chances and have her uterus removed and preserves both the ovaries. It was decided to perform VH and preserve both the ovaries.[3,12,22] There was no indication to use a laparoscope or fallaciously open the abdomen.[22-28]
Diagnosis: CIN III
Operation: VH

Vaginal hysterectomy was performed as per routine but along with a vaginal cuff of 3 cm including 1 cm below the fornix (Fig. 1). Cut open uterus showed normal endometrium and endocervix with adenomyotic uterine walls. Unhealthy cervix but not cancerous looking on naked eye examination. Tubes and ovaries were healthy. Prophylactic bilateral salpingectomy was performed[29] and healthy ovaries preserved (age: 43 years). After checking hemostasis, closure was done. Blood transfusion was not needed. Hospital stay was 36 hours. Postoperatively she had an uneventful speedy recovery.
Histopathology: It showed uterus weighed 120 g with moderate adenomyosis, normal tubes and CIN III of cervix

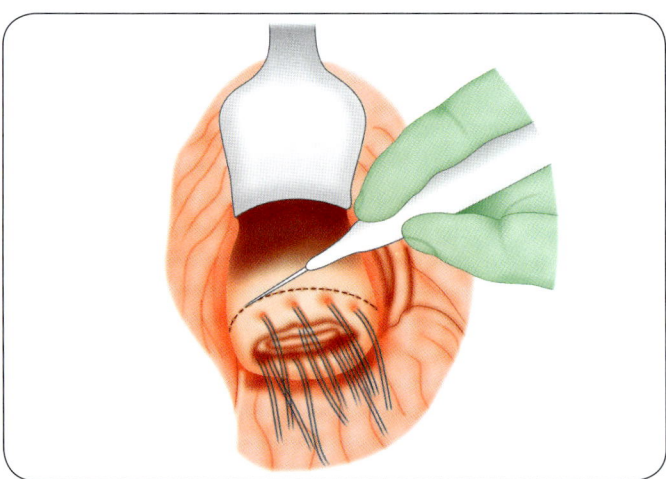

Fig. 1: The incision is continued anteriorly around the entire circumference of the vagina, taking care not to injure the bladder.
Source: In: Rock JA, Thompson JD (Eds). TeLinde's Operative Gynecology, 8th edition. Philadelphia, PA, USA: Lippincott-Raven Publishers; 1997. pp. 1413-99.

without the slightest doubt. HP slides were double checked by taking a second opinion of a reputed pathologist.

Performing laparoscopic hysterectomy for CIN III is like performing for cervical erosion or DUB of the past and worse would be to open the abdomen for it. This is essential for oncosurgeons, particularly gyneco-oncosurgeons to note and routinely advise VH for CIN III and not give disadvantageous treatment or call themselves gyneconcosurgeons.
What inspired: Premalignant condition.

LESSONS

- VH is ideal for not uncommon CIN III.
- It is ideal to take a second opinion of a reputed pathologist on the HP slides of the preoperative cervical biopsy as well as the postoperatively removed organ, when diagnosis deals with cancer.

CASE 69: VH FOR METASTATIC BREAST CANCER PLUS UTERINE ADENOMYOSIS

Name: Mrs. X
Age: 57 years
Parity: 3 FTND
LD: 30 years back
H/O: Left mastectomy—2 years back for "Breast Cancer (CA)" (Figs. 1 and 2) followed by chemotherapy, tamoxifen etc.

Clinically 8-week size uterus with free mobility. Cervix with simple erosion on both the lips with physiological descent to attempt VH and clear fornices.

Sonography: It revealed uterus volume 110 cm^3, adenomyotic with 4 mm endometrial thickness and clear fornices.

Her oncosurgeon was keen to have bilateral oophorectomy for which she was referred.

She was explained the pros and cons in detail about uterine conservation versus removal and also the need for regular "Pap" smear, like anyone else. After preoperative counseling, she expressed her desire to have slightly enlarged uterus also removed along with ovaries as she had menorrhagia in past and unlikely to do a "Pap" test on a regular basis. In other words, to have BSO plus hysterectomy.

It was decided to perform VH plus BSO as there was no contraindication or finding to dissuade it.[30-33]

Diagnosis: Breast cancer with uterine adenomyosis.
Operation: VH with prophylactic BSO.

Vaginal hysterectomy plus BSO performed as per routine without any difficulty. Hemostasis was checked and vaginal closure done. Blood transfusion was not needed. Hospital stay was 2 days. Postoperatively she had an uneventful speedy recovery. HP showed uterus of 130 g with moderate adenomyosis. Right ovary showed benign adenofibroma. Tubes and ovaries were otherwise normal. No malignancy.

She was referred back or handed over to oncosurgeon for her future breast cancer-related management.
What inspired: Indication for bilateral oophorectomy.

LESSON

- If breast cancer indicates bilateral oophorectomy[3,32,33] and if gynecologically uterus merits removal, it is worth taking the vaginal route for VH plus BSO and give benefits out of it.

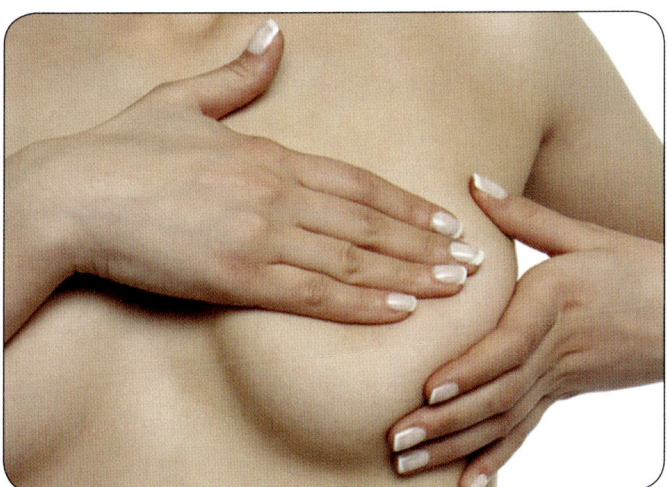

Fig. 1: On palpation, feels firm area needing clinical examination and mammography.

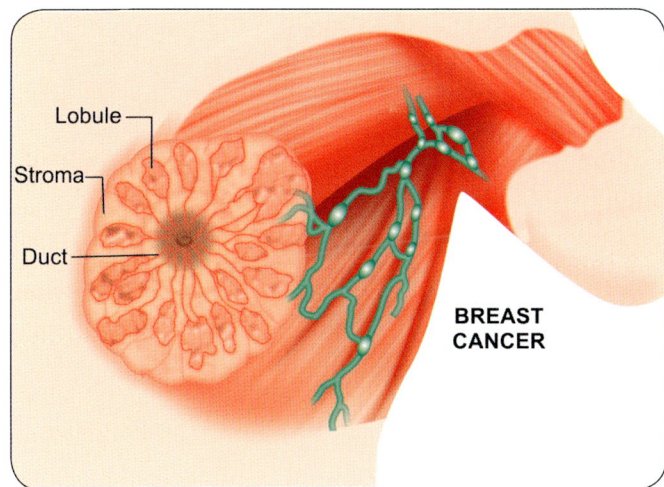

Fig. 2: Breast cancer.

CASE 70: VH: PROPHYLACTIC FOR HYDATIDIFORM MOLE

Name: Mrs. X
Age: 39 years
Parity: 2 FTND
LD: 10 years back

She had 3 months amenorrhea, 18-week size uterus with absent external ballottement and fetal heart sounds. Blood beta-human chorionic gonadotropin (β-hCG) level was above 100,000, and sonography confirmed the diagnosis of molar pregnancy. She was 39 years old with two children, wanting tubal sterilization, i.e. no more pregnancy.

She was explained the pros and cons of molar pregnancy and resultant trophoblastic malignancy[34] including selectively prophylactic chemotherapy or even hysterectomy.

She was keen to have a hysterectomy and take no risk in the future. Choice was between:
- Laparoscopic hysterectomy/LAVH
- Abdominal hysterectomy
- VH.

If VH, it should be attempted only after uterine evacuation as uterus of 18+ weeks size with volume of 600+ cm^3 can give excessive intra- and postevacuational bleeding.

Hysterectomy can be undertaken soon after the uterine evacuation is complete, i.e. at the same sitting or alternatively 6–8 weeks later after the uterine involution. Latter has risk of woman changing her mind and may prefer not to undergo prophylactic hysterectomy. After necessary counseling, it was decided and advised to first have uterine evacuation, followed by hysterectomy via vaginal route.[34,35]

Diagnosis: Hydatidiform mole (vesicular mole).
Operation: Prophylactic VH.
What deters/dissuades: Enlarged vascular, soft uterus.

She had uterine evacuation by suction curettage with intravenous drip of 5% dextrose containing oxytocin and keeping blood units available as her Hb% was 10.5 g. Soft and vascular uterus almost became 14 weeks size after evacuation. Saline adrenaline infiltration at the start, gentleness and extra care was exercised during hysterectomy. Hysterectomy was performed by standard technique without the slightest difficulty. In fact, planes of cleavage and access to the peritoneum were easier. Normal tubes and ovaries were preserved as per preoperative counseling and informed consent. Hemostasis was checked and vaginal closure done. Hospital stay was 2 days with an uneventful postoperative speedy recovery. Follow-up showed decline of β-hCG level and return to normal.

Histopathology: It showed enlarged uterus of 290 g with thick vascular uterine walls, fair amount of vesicles and clots in the uterine cavity. No malignancy.

Uterus differs from routine gynecological uteri, as it gets debulked in size by evacuation of the contents just as uterus becomes smaller after delivering a fetus. Debulking is without the use of a knife.

Advantage is great as VH is the least invasive and advantageous when compared with the alternative techniques for hysterectomy. It is economical with better outcome and fewer complications. Hysterectomy will take away risk of trophoblastic malignancy or other aftermath.

What inspired: Need for prophylactic hysterectomy.

LESSON

- When required, can choose vaginal route for prophylactic hysterectomy in women with or without H/O hydatidiform mole.[35]

CASE 71: VH WITH BSO FOR TWISTED OVARIAN CYST

Name: Mrs. X
Age: 52 years
Parity: 4 FTND
LD: 22 years back.
C/O: Severe lower abdominal pain, vomiting.
Last menstrual period (LMP): 4 years back.

Mildly obese (BMI 32), mild hypertension and no diabetes. Tachycardia, lower abdominal tenderness, guarding and mild distension present. Clinically uterus normal size with restricted mobility. Normal cervix showed physiological descent to attempt hysterectomy. Left and posterior fornices filled with tender, cystic mass.

Sonography: It showed uterine volume of 50 cm³ with left ovarian cyst in pouch of Douglas (POD) 9 × 5 × 4.6 cm, hemorrhagic with clots, without any septa and solid area with twists, reported as left twisted ovarian cyst by a reliable sonologist Dr Darshana Kshirsagar, Consultant Radiologist, NM Medical Center, Mumbai, India. Right tube and ovary were normal. Preoperative diagnosis was twisted left ovarian cyst with acute abdomen. Preoperative work out was normal.

Treatment needed and advised was hysterectomy with BSO. Twisted ovarian cyst per se demands laparoscopic surgery or laparotomy, and vaginal route is not ever considered or mentioned in the literature for its management.[36-38]

However, on assessing her for VH, clinically cervix and uterus were favorable for hysterectomy. Moot question then was of dealing with 'Twisted ovarian cyst'. Past experience of salpingo-oophorectomy for adnexal pathology including some not so easy and experience of only one case of twisted ovarian cyst dealt vaginally, encouraged and inspired to undertake vaginal route.[39]

Diagnosis: Left twisted ovarian cyst.
Operation: VH with BSO. 'Trial Vaginal Route'.
What deters/dissuades vaginal route: Twisted ovarian cyst and emergency.

Clinically and examination under anesthesia favored VH. Taken as 'Trial Vaginal Route' case.[3,5] VH was straightforward. After uterines were secured as the cyst was on the left side, all lateral connections, including cornual or upper pedicle, were excised on the right side to free the uterus on the right side. Thus, the freed uterus from its connections on the right was turned to the left so that the posterior uterine surface faced the operator. This gave ample free space to visualize the contents in POD and make ovary and tube free from surrounding adhesions. After safe isolation of the operative field all-round by covering the area with an isolation sheet, cyst was punctured with 16 No. needle to

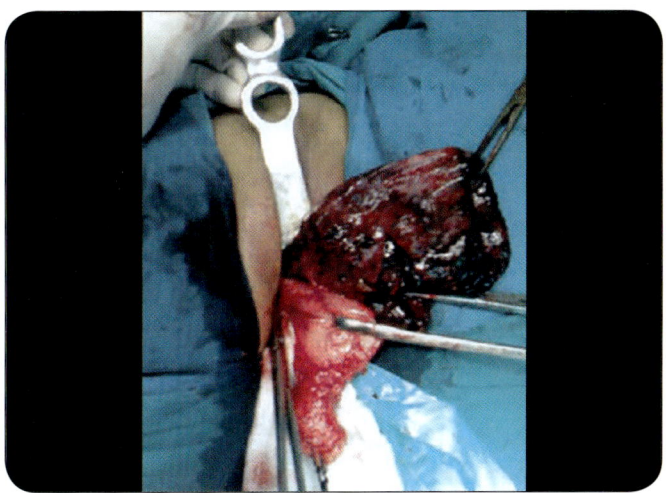

Fig. 1: Twisted ovarian cyst. Uterus with severed left lateral connections and intact right upper pedicle showing a debulked, gangrenous and necrotic ovarian cyst measuring 10.5 cm, 8.5 cm and 8.6 cm[38]

debulk the cyst and get it exteriorized. Needle was connected to a suction apparatus. 265 cc of hemorrhagic fluid was easily aspirated. Gravity from head-high position, suprapubic pressure and gentle traction on the free uterus to the left showed gangrenous, necrotic, hemorrhagic cyst on the left with two twists at infundibulopelvic ligament (IPL). Left round ligament was cut as distally or laterally as possible to get an access to IPL and clamp it for salpingo-oophorectomy, which included twisted gangrenous cystic mass. This was easily possible. It was then followed by prophylactic salpingo-oophorectomy of contralateral normal right tube and ovary, so as to have BSO. This had earlier been consented to by the patient. Cut open uterus showed normal endometrial lining. Blood transfusion was not needed. Hospital stay was 2 days followed by an uneventful speedy recovery (Fig. 1).

Histopathology: It showed typical of twisted cyst, totally infracted and gangrenous, reddish brown, hemorrhagic, necrotic collapsed benign cyst along with left tube and left ovary. Uterus, right tube and ovary were normal. No malignancy.

What inspired: (1) Major parameters were normal for possible VH and (2) Back up experience of salpingo-oophorectomy for adnexal pathology at VH.

Crux: Zeal and enthusiasm for rare attempt.

LESSONS

- Inspiring to recommend to experienced colleagues, when an opportunity arises.
- Zeal and enthusiasm gave benefits.

CASE 72: VH FOR UTERINE FIBROIDS WITH H/O FAILED ABDOMINAL HYSTERECTOMY

Name: Mrs. X
Age: 34 years
H/O: Multiple myomectomies abdominally in 1989.

She remained asymptomatic for 18 months after myomectomies in the past but had recurrence of fibroids including submucous one with resultant menorrhagia. Medical treatment failed and she opted for hysterectomy. In fact, she was keen to have her uterus out. Unfortunately in 1991, abdominal hysterectomy failed as the operator, a colleague in Mumbai, could not gain access to the pelvic cavity and so reach the fundus, tubes and ovaries. Intestines and omentum were adherent to the abdominal wall and attempts to separate them failed. Hysterectomy was abandoned and the abdomen closed by the operating gynecologist.

In 1996, there was continuous bleeding for 6 weeks for which treatment and further feasible action was needed. The author was consulted for the first time. Clinical examination showed 12 weeks, nodular uterus with slightly restricted mobility, normal cervix with physiological descent to attempt VH. Lateral fornices were clear and there was no contraindication to VH. Sonography showed that uterus volume 260 cm³ with fibroids.[40] Tubes and ovaries appeared normal. She was taken as "Trial VH as well as Trial Vaginal Route"[3,5] with surgeon's availability, if intestinal surgery was required, i.e. standby with facilities for laparotomy.

Vaginal hysterectomy was chosen as: (1) Clinical and pelvic findings during examination under anesthesia showed that the anterior as well as the posterior cul-de-sac should be accessible and there was a freely mobile uterus and favorable descent of normal cervix. (2) The uterine size was not unduly large and it was debulkable.[22] In case, there were flimsy adhesions they could be lysed via the vaginal route.[3] Cohen[41] writes that the viscera above the uterus might have even cobwebs and dense adhesions, but the uterus felt vaginally can be totally free. This is a very inspiring and vital observation. Therefore, if surrounding organs were protected from the trauma, the uterus can just slip out. The patient was fully counseled about possible failure of the VH and then the need of alternative measures, such as a change to abdominal hysterectomy. She was also informed that hysterectomy by either route can badly traumatize the intestines, bladder and rectum and in the event of such complications, a general surgeon was needed to be available to take over. She was warned that if that happened, there might be a long hospital stay and another procedure (i.e. closure of colostomy) might be necessary 6–8 weeks later.[42] She freely consented for it (Figs. 1 and 2).

Diagnosis: Uterine fibroids with H/O failed abdominal hysterectomy.
Operation: VH.
What deters/dissuades: Failed abdominal hysterectomy and now if VH fails.

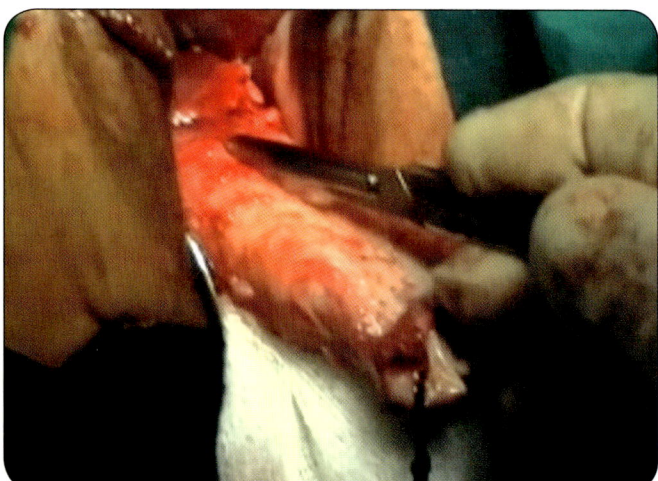

Fig. 1: After uterine vessels are secured, cervix is bisected to reach uterine cavity for the fibroid or its bulge.

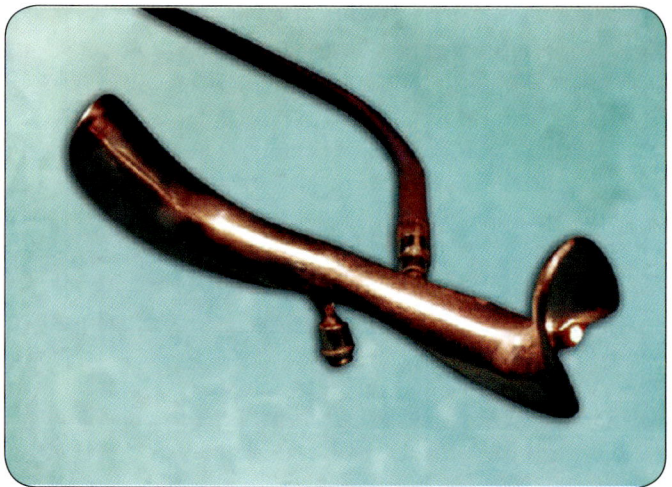

Fig. 2: Sim's vaginal speculum with fiberoptic light facility.[43]

Cervical descent was adequate to start VH and continue. Access to POD was not difficult. Cervix and further lower uterus bisected to enucleate fibroids and adenomyotic uterine walls from inside keeping serosa intact. Hysterectomy was interestingly straightforward and flimsy adhesions near the fundus and upper part of the uterine body were easily dealt with. Adhesions between the uterine fundus and bowel were carefully separated. Fiberoptic light was useful for distal approach.[43] Thus, hysterectomy was completed without any damage or trauma to neighboring organs/tissues. Tubes and ovaries were normal. They were preserved (age: 34 years). Nothing distally required to be explored. Blood loss was less than 100 mL. Hemostasis was checked and vaginal closure done. Blood transfusion was not needed. Fortunately, there was no need to access the abdomen or ask for the help of a surgeon.

Surgeon was most sincerely thanked for his availability and providing assurance. She was discharged after 2 days of surgery and had an uneventful speedy recovery.

Histopathology: It showed uterus weighted 280 g with fibroids and moderate adenomyosis. No malignancy.

Alternatives were:
- Transcervical resection of endometrium (TCRE) i.e. endometrial ablation or use intrauterine long acting device.
- Attempt to repeat abdominal hysterectomy
- Laparoscopic hysterectomy, if possible by a highly experienced laparoscopic surgeon
- Radiotherapy, though undesirable
- Venture to attempt VH
- The question asked for decision making was: "With the same clinical findings in absence of previously failed abdominal surgery, though rare, would I have subjected her to hysterectomy via the vaginal route?" The answer was "yes" or favorable. It was worth going ahead with necessary precautions. Surely repeat abdominal hysterectomy can be more risky than attempting VH.

What inspired:
- Favorable clinical and under anesthesia pelvic findings
- Cohen's[41] observation, mentioned in his book.

LESSON

- Zeal and enthusiasm on the part of the gynecologist can help to give huge relief to the patient.

CASE 73: VH UNDER LOCAL ANESTHESIA FOR PULMONARY FIBROSIS

Name: Mrs. X
Age: 64 years
Parity: 3 FTND
LMP: 9 years back
C/O: Postmenopausal bleeding.

The patient had a H/O hysteroscopy plus D&C with endometrial HP showing complex hyperplasia with atypia (no malignancy). Clinically the uterus was of 8 weeks size, healthy cervix with physiological descent and clear fornices. Sonography showed a uterus of 130 cm³ volume with normal pelvic findings.

She was a known case of pulmonary fibrosis with a need for continuous therapeutic oxygen. Laparoscopic hysterectomy or abdominal hysterectomy was contraindicated and there was a very high-risk. Colleagues at major hospitals had declined to operate. After necessary evaluation and consultations with the chest physician and anesthesiologist, it was decided to perform VH under local anesthesia. Surgery was essential as cytologic atypia with complex hyperplasia has a 23% risk of developing endometrial malignancy.[44]

The decision to operate under local anesthesia was carefully discussed with the patient and relatives at length and also with the anesthesiologist, who agreed to supplement it, if required. Well-informed consent was taken before attempting VH under local anesthesia.[45]

Diagnosis: Endometrial complex hyperplasia with atypia plus pulmonary fibrosis.

Operation: VH under local anesthesia.

What deters/dissuades VH: Local anesthesia failure.

In the past, the patient used to be premedicated with 50+ mg intravenously (IV) meperidine plus 25 mg promethazine hydrochloride intramuscularly 30 minutes before surgery. An additional IV infusion of 500 mL 5% D/W (5% dextrose in water) containing 100 mg meperidine was administered very slowly as decided by the attending anesthesiologist.

At present, one uses lorazepam (ativan) 1 mg HS, then 45 minutes before surgery, injection butorphanol 1 mg intramuscularly plus promethazine 25 mg 45–60 minutes before surgery. Injection clonidine 0.5 mg/kg intramuscularly can also be used 30 minutes before surgery. Currently options are many. This followed by careful induction with benzodiazepine-midazolam 0.05–0.10 mg/kg IV plus opioid (fentanyl) 2 µg/kg IV and propofol 1.5–2 mg/kg IV and maintain with gas plus oxygen plus volatile anesthesia agent.

She was placed in the lithotomy position and prepared for surgery only after she was well sedated. For this surgery, patients should be drowsy and should not move on insertion of the vaginal speculum. Pudendal and paracervical nerve blocks were given with a 1% solution of lidocaine hydrochloride. About 25 mL was used for the pudendal block and 10 mL for the paracervical block. Care was taken not to exceed a total of 40 mL (Figs. 1 and 2).

The need was to be as gentle as possible with the tissues. This was facilitated by performing clampless hysterectomy which the author does routinely.[46,47] Lighter and smaller instruments were used for vaginal wall retraction. When the patient perceived a dragging or disturbing pain, a small amount of additional local infiltration was done. From time to time, vocal reassurance by the anesthetist and when required, additional local infiltration helped. Once the uterus was removed, hemostasis was checked and vaginal closure done. Salpingo-oophorectomy was not done as there was no family H/O ovarian malignancy and patient was not keen to have it.

Blood transfusion was not needed. Hospital stay was 4 days; the extra day was due to the pulmonary status. She made an uneventful recovery.

On HP, the uterus weighed 140 g with complex hyperplasia, marked atypia and no malignancy.

Some women who require a hysterectomy may have medical problems that do not permit the safe administration of either general or regional anesthesia. Local anesthesia was uncommonly used in the past in high-risk patients to perform VH. Only those women who are assessed as being highly cooperative should be considered for surgery under local anesthesia. An anesthesiologist must always be present for continuous intraoperative monitoring throughout the surgery.

Conventionally, major gynecologic surgery is performed under either general anesthesia or regional anesthesia. Although this is suitable for the vast majority, there are some high-risk patients with coexisting medical disease contraindicating such anesthesia. Gynecologists are sometimes forced to cancel surgeries because of the anesthesiologist

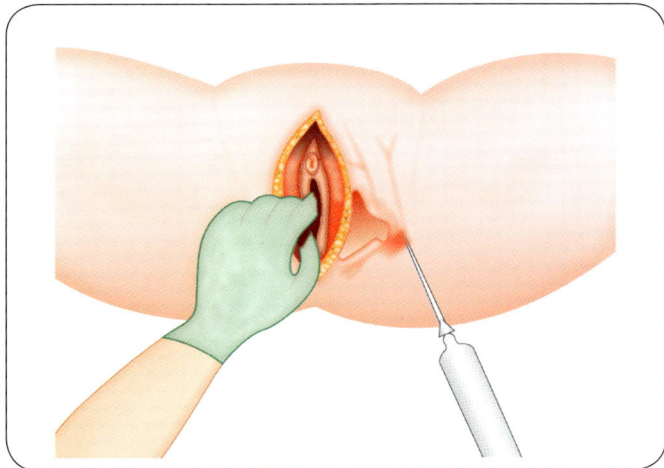

Fig. 1: Pudendal block for anesthesia of the perineum.

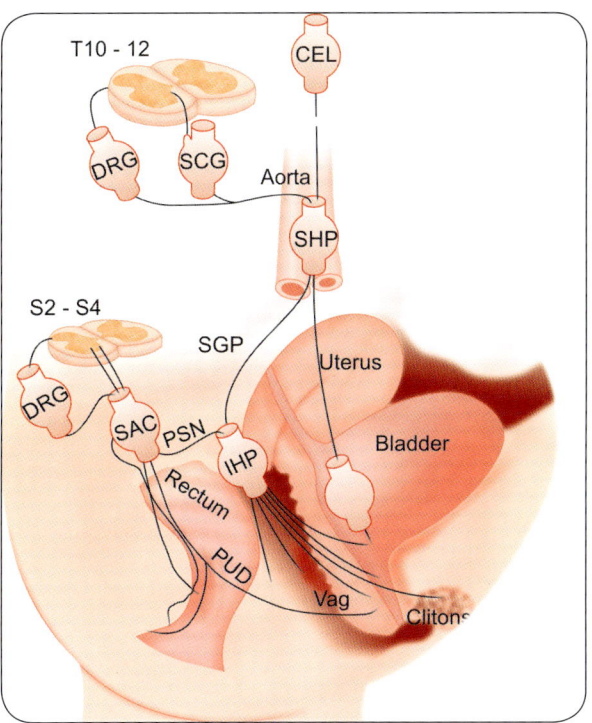

Fig. 2: Illustration of the innervation of the pelvis. The superior hypogastric plexus is excised during a presacral neurectomy.
Source: In: Gomel V, Brill AI (Eds). Reconstructive and Reproductive Surgery in Gynecology. London, UK: Informa Health Care; 2010. pp. 138-56.

declining to give anesthesia in the best interests of the patients. Ischemic heart disease with low ejection fraction or extensive lung disease (chronic obstructive pulmonary disease), or malnourished and debilitated patients are not uncommon in our population and are the largest group of such patients.

The use of local anesthesia for performing gynecologic surgery was emphasized to appreciate the number of advantages local anesthesia offers.[48] Decades ago Gellhorn[49] used preliminary twilight sleep and parametrial infiltration to perform VH in 82 women. Ramos et al.[50] performed VH with repair in 27 women between the ages of 51 years and 83 years with genital prolapse under local anesthesia, supplemented occasionally with IV sodium pentothal. Of course, now facilities have changed drastically to make previously unsafe conditions safe for anesthesia. When few anesthesiologists were on leave for the postgraduate examinations, at KEM Hospital and Seth GS Medical College, Mumbai, India, I had the pleasure of gaining experience of performing vaginal hysterectomies under local anesthesia instead of postponing them.[45]

What inspired: Not to postpone in the interest of the patient. Learning to do so.

LESSONS

- Familiarity with the techniques of pudendal block, paracervical block and local infiltration adds to the technique and armamentarium under compelling conditions
- When needed, local anesthesia can come to the rescue of such patients and their gynecologists, provided an anesthesiologist is part of the team.

CASE 74: VH WITH ALTERED APPROACH TO VUP (VH WITH BSO)

Name: Mrs. X
Age: 62 years
Parity: 3 FTND
H/O: No relevant history
   Not obese but hypertensive without H/O diabetes.
   Clinically uterus normal size with third-degree uterine prolapse. Moderate cystocele and rectocele. No stress urinary incontinence.
Sonography: It revealed uterine volume 46 cm³ with elongated cervix. Tubes and ovaries were normal.
Diagnosis: Third-degree uterine prolapse with cystocele and rectocele.
Operation: VH with BSO plus anterior colporrhaphy and posterior colpoperineorrhaphy.

Vaginal hysterectomy started as usual except anterior vaginal incision was at a much higher level, closer to the urethral meatus and away from the external os because of elongated cervix. Bladder separation was attempted carefully but it could not be adequately separated to see or feel vesicouterine peritoneum (VUP). Posterior cul-de-sac was easily accessed and uterosacrals and Mackendrot's ligaments and uterine vessels secured. This permitted to apply Allis' forceps to posterior uterine wall from pouch of Douglas (POD) and give a gentle traction to bring out the uterine fundus from posterior and exposing anterior uterine surface. This happened easily from the posterior space, showing a drooping bladder below anterior uterocervical junction (Fig. 1). Babcock was put on the bladder and VUP was carefully incised.[4] From the incised area, a finger was inserted from posterior to anterior. This showed thin peritoneum covering the inserted finger. Peritoneum was then cut and widened to insert the bladder retractor. Rest of the surgery was done as required, i.e.

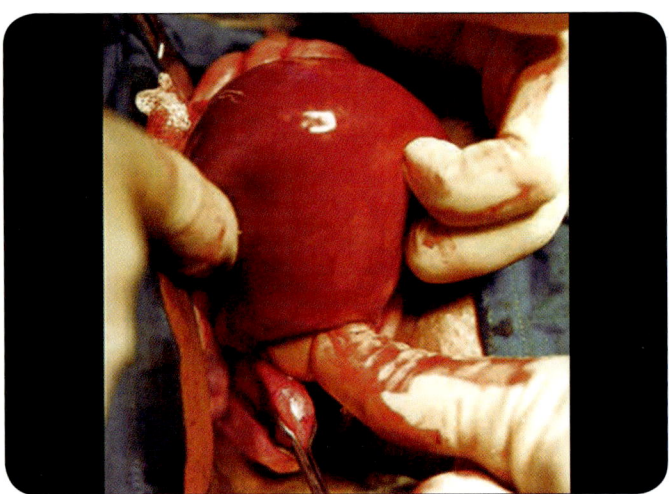

Fig. 1: Uterine fundus is delivered from the posterior pouch of Douglas (POD) and pulled in front. Babcock's forceps clearly show the bladder and site of vesicouterine peritoneum (VUP) to be accessed—the reverse of what is done at abdominal hysterectomy for similar access.[4]

VH with BSO plus anterior colporrhaphy and posterior colpoperineorrhaphy repair. Hemostasis was checked and vaginal closure done. Blood transfusion was not needed. Hospital stay was 2 days as patient preferred to go home with a self-retaining catheter. Catheter was removed on 5th morning by a nurse sent to the patient's home. She made an uneventful recovery.

Histopathology: It showed uterus weighing 50 g with atrophic endometrium. Tubes and ovaries were without pathology. No malignancy.

LESSON

- VUP accessed from the posterior to tackle the bladder separation.

CASE 75: VH WITH BICORNUATE UTERUS

Name: Mrs. X
Age: 48 years
Parity: 1 FTCS
H/O: No relevant history
C/O: Heavy menses for 1 year.
Not obese with no H/O hypertension or diabetes.
Clinically uterus 10 weeks size, healthy cervix with physiological descent and clear fornices.
Sonography: It revealed uterine volume 190 cm^3 with few fibroids and endometrial thickness 14 mm. Tubes and ovaries were normal. Bicornuate uterus was diagnosed earlier at caesarean section.
Diagnosis: Uterine fibroids with bicornuate uterus (Fig. 1).
Operation: VH.
What deters/dissuades: Combination of caesarean section and bicornuate uterus.

Vaginal hysterectomy started by approaching utero-cervical-broad ligament space to separate the bladder. It needed much more separation as higher up the uterus was broad to fully accommodate the posterior surface of the bladder. Careful separation was easy to show thin peritoneum. After uterines were secured, uterus was mildly debulked to confirm that uterus is bicornuate. Hysterectomy completed by severance of lateral pedicles, very close to lateral uterine walls. After checking hemostasis, vaginal closure was done. Blood transfusion was not needed.

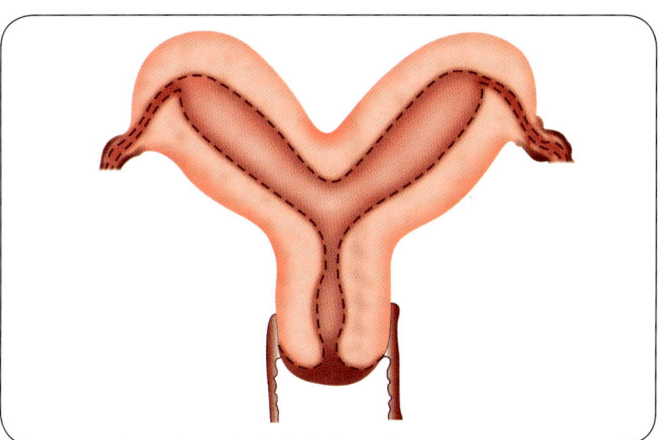

Fig. 1: A bicornuate uterus.[51]

Hospital stay was 2 days. Postoperatively she had an uneventful speedy recovery.
Histopathology: It showed uterus was typically bicornuate, weighed 205 g and severe adenomyosis with few fibroids. Tubes and ovaries were normal. No malignancy.
What inspired: Bicornuate uterus.

LESSON

- Bicornuate uterus should never inhibit vaginal route or cause anxiety. In fact adds flavor.

CASE 76: BLADDER STONE REMOVAL AT VH PLUS ANTERIOR AND POSTERIOR REPAIR

Name: Mrs. X
Age: 48 years
Parity: 3 FTND
C/O: Something coming down per vaginam, hematuria and colicky—spasmodic lower abdominal pain attacks. Not obese with no H/O hypertension or diabetes.

Clinically uterus was 6 weeks size with third-degree uterine prolapse and cysto-rectoceles. Systemic findings were normal.

Sonography: Normal abdominopelvic findings. Uterine volume was 30 cm^3 with normal adnexa. Additionally, vesical stones of 5 cm × 3 cm, 4 cm × 2 cm and two small ones. Preoperatively, other investigations were normal. For her bladder stones, she was counseled that stones can be freely and safely taken out during vaginal surgery by opening the bladder instead of similar surgery via abdominal route (or at another session). Abdomen will be thus kept intact. Postoperatively, she will have urinary catheter in the bladder for 7–10 days.

Diagnosis: Third-degree uterine prolapse, moderate cystocele, mild rectocele and multiple vesical calculi.

Operation: VH, cystotomy, anterior colporrhaphy and posterior colpoperineorrhaphy.

What deters/dissuades: Distance at which ureters are.

Vaginal hysterectomy done as per routine. Normal tubes and ovaries were preserved. Then after, bladder was held carefully and opened safely. Stones were removed or taken out and saline lavage given before its closure in three layers. At this stage, one felt gratified as woman was spared from abdominal access. This was followed by required anterior colporrhaphy as if bladder has remained untouched and thenafter it was followed by posterior colpoperineorrhaphy. Self retaining catheter was kept in to rest the bladder and permit healing for 10 days. She had no difficulty in passing urine on her own with residual urine of less than 10 cc. Hospital stay was for 11 days as at home she would be uncomfortable and apprehensive with urinary catheter. Postoperative period was uneventful with speed recovery.

Histopathology: It showed uterus weighed 36 g with no abnormality. No malignancy.

What inspired: Uterine prolapse with cystocele.

LESSON

- Can spare abdominal approach for vesical calculi and related postoperative care. Minus side is gynecologist removing bladder stones and ethics. Had such a case many years back.

REFERENCES

1. Sheth SS. Results of treatment of rupture of the uterus by suturing. J Obstet Gynecol of Brit Commonwealth. 1968; 75:55-8.
2. Sheth SS. Suturing of the tear as treatment in uterine rupture. Am J Obstet Gynecol. 1969;105(3):440-3.
3. Sheth SS, Paghdiwalla KP, Hajari AR. Vaginal route: A gynaecological route for much more than hysterectomy. Best Pract Res Clin Obstet Gynaecol. 2011;25(2):115-32.
4. Sheth SS. Access to vesicouterine and rectouterine pouches. In: Sheth SS (Ed). Vaginal Hysterectomy, 2nd edition. New Delhi, India: Jaypee Brothers Medical Publishers (P) Ltd; 2014. pp. 31-50.
5. Sheth SS. Vaginal hysterectomy. In: Studd J (Ed). Progress in Obstetrics and Gynecology, 10th edition. London, UK: Churchill Livingstone; 1993. pp. 317-40.
6. Sheth SS. Vaginal hysterectomy following earlier ruptured uterus and caesarean sections. J Gynecol Surg. 1998;14:185-9.
7. Sheth SS, Malpani AN. Vaginal hysterectomy following previous caesarean section. Int. J Gynecol Obstet. 1995;50(2): 165-9.
8. Sheth SS. An approach to vesicouterine peritoneum through a new surgical space. J Gynecol Surg. 1996;12:135-40.
9. Sizzi O, Paparella P, Bonito C, Paparella R, Rossetti A. Laparoscopic assistance after vaginal hysterectomy and unsuccessful access to the ovaries or failed uterine mobilization: changing trends. JSLS. 2004;8(4):339-46.
10. Monaghan JM. *Personal communication*.
11. Khung TT. Use of Sheth's uterocervical broad ligament space for vaginal hysterectomy in a patient with history of caesarean section. Malaysian J of Obstet Gynaecol. 1995;4 (1-2):39-42.
12. Sheth SS, Paghdiwalla K. Do we need the laparoscopic route? J Obstet Gynaecol India. 2001;51:25-30.
13. Kovac SR, Cruiskshank SH, Retto HF. Laparoscopy-assisted vaginal hysterectomy. J Gynecol Surg. 1990;6:185-92.
14. Coulam CB, Pratt JH. Vaginal hysterectomy. Is previous pelvic operation a contraindication? Am J Obstet Gynecol. 1973;116:252-60.
15. Sheth SS. Broad ligament myomectomy at vaginal hysterectomy without laparoscopic assistance. J Gynecol Surg. 2007;23:133-42.

16. Sheth SS. A surgical window to access the obliterated posterior cul-de-sac at vaginal hysterectomy. Int J Gynecol Obstet. 2009;107:244-7.
17. Sheth SS. Adnexectomy for benign pathology at vaginal hysterectomy without laparoscopic assistance. Br J Obstet Gynecol. 2002;109:1401-5.
18. Sheth SS. Newer perspectives. In: Sheth SS (Ed). Vaginal Hysterectomy, 2nd edition. New Delhi, India: Jaypee Brothers Medical Publishers (P) Ltd; 2014. pp. 225-34.
19. Macleod D, Howkins J (Eds). Hysterectomy for cervical and broad ligament myoma. In: Bonney's Gynaecological Surgery, 7th edition. London, UK: William Clowes and Sons, Ltd.; 1964. pp. 253-76.
20. Edozien LC. Hysterectomy for benign conditions. BMJ. 2005;330:1457.
21. Sheth SS, Rathi MR. Uterine fibroids. In: Sheth SS (Ed). Vaginal Hysterectomy, 2nd edition. New Delhi, India: Jaypee Brothers Medical Publishers (P) Ltd; 2014. pp. 72-89.
22. Sheth SS. Vaginal or abdominal hysterectomy. In: Sheth SS (Ed). Vaginal Hysterectomy, 2nd edition. New Delhi, India: Jaypee Brothers Medical Publishers (P) Ltd; 2014. pp. 273-93.
23. Morrow CP. In: Mishell DR, Kirschbaum RH, Morrow CP (Eds). Year Book of Obstetrics, Gynecology and Operative Gynecology. St. Louis: Mosby; 1994. pp. 257-83.
24. Van der Stege JG, Van Beek JJ. Problems rela.0ted to the cervical stump at follow-up in laparoscopic supracervical hysterectomy. J Soc Laparoendoscopic Surgeons. 1999;3:5-7.
25. Sheth SS. Vaginal excision of cervical stump. J Obstet Gynecol. 2000;20:523-4.
26. Epithelial abnormalities of the genital tract. In: Kumar P, Malhotra N (Eds). Jeffcott's Principles of Gynaecology, 7th international edition. New Delhi, India: Jaypee Brothers Medical Publishers (P) Ltd; 2008. pp. 400-26.
27. Jones HW. Cervical cancer precursors and their management. In: Rock JA, Jones HW (Eds). TeLinde's Operative Gynecology, Volume 2, 10th edition. Philadelphia, PA, USA: Lippincott Williams & Wilkins; 2008. pp. 1208-26.
28. Miskry T, Magos A, Subtotal vaginal hysterectomy. In: Sheth SS (Ed). Vaginal Hysterectomy, 2nd edition. New Delhi, India: Jaypee Brothers Medical Publishers (P) Ltd; 2014. pp. 163-71.
29. Kwon JS, Tinker A, Pansegrau G, et al. Prophylactic salpingectomy and delayed oophorectomy as an alternative for BRCA mutation carriers. Obstet Gynecol. 2013;121:14-24.
30. Sheth SS. Vaginal route for breast cancer induced hysterectomy with oophorectomy. J obstet Gynecol. 2011;31:533-4.
31. Sheth SS. Vaginal Oophorectomy for breast cancer. J Obstet Gynecol. 1989;9:236-8.
32. Adanu RM, Hammoud MM. Contemporary issues in women's health. Int J Obstet Gynecol. 2010;109:3-4.
33. ACOG Today. Vaginal hysterectomy often better option than abdominal. Am Coll Obstet Gynecol Bull. 2009;14.
34. Cunningham FG, Lenevo KJ, Bloom SL, Hauth JC, Gilstrap LC III, Wenstrom KD, Gestational trophoblastic disease (Eds.). Williams Obstetrics, International edition (22nd edition). USA: McGraw-Hill Companies; 2005. pp. 273-84.
35. Sheth SS. Prophylactic vaginal hysterectomy for benign hydatidiform mole. Int J Gynaecol Obstet. 2007;96(1):38-9.
36. Mage G, Canis M, Manhes H, Pouly JL, Bruhat MA. Laparoscopic management of adnexal torsion. A review of 35 cases. J Reprod Med. 1989;34:520-4.
37. Shalev E, Peleg D. Laparoscopic treatment of adnexal torsion. Surg Gynecol Obstet. 1993;176:448-50.
38. Cohen SB, Wattiez A, Seidman DS, et al. Laparoscopy versus laparotomy for detorsion and sparing of twisted ischemic adnexa. JSLS. 2003;7:295-9.
39. Sheth SS, Sriinivasan R, Darda P. Twisted ovarian cyst treated via the vaginal route. Inj J Gynecol Obstet. 2011;113:245-6.
40. Sheth SS, Shah NM. Preoperative sonographic estimation of uterine volume: an aid to determine the route of hysterectomy. J Gynecol Surg. 2002;18:13-22.
41. Cohen J. Abdominal and Vaginal Hysterectomy: New Techniques Based on Time and Motion Studies, 1st edition. London, UK: Heinemann Medical; 1972. pp. 72-132.
42. Sheth SS, Goyal MV, Sheth J, Navle V. Vaginal hysterectomy following failed abdominal hysterectomy. J Gynecol Surg. 1998;14:191-3.
43. Sheth SS. Fiberoptic light for oophorectomy at vaginal hysterectomy. Obstet Gynecol Surv. 1999;54:171-2.
44. Kurman RJ, Kaminski PF, Norris HJ. The behavior of endometrial hyperplasia: a long-term study of "untreated" hyperplasia in 170 patients. Cancer. 1985;56:403.
45. Sheth SS, Malpani A, Vaginal hysterectomy for high-risk patients under local anesthesia. J Gynecol Surg. 1992;8:65-7.
46. Halban J. Gynakologische operations. Lehre, Vienna, Urban & Schwarzenberg, 1932, cited in Falk HC, Soichet S. The technique of vaginal hysterectomy. Clin Obstet Gynecol. 1972;15:703.
47. Sheth SS. Vaginal hysterectomy. Best Pract Res Clin Obstet Gynaecol. 2005;19(3):307-32.
48. Penfield AJ. Gynecologic Surgery Under Local Anesthesia. Baltimore: Urban & Schwarzenberg; 1988.
49. Gelhorn G. Vaginal hysterectomy under local anesthesia. Surg Gynecol Obstet. 1930;51:484.
50. Ramos P, Alberto G, Goni M. Vaginal hysterectomy for genital prolapse of elderly women. Bol Soc Obstet Ginecol Buenos Aires. 1954;33:407.
51. Rock JA. Surgery for anomalies of the Mullerian ducts. In: Rock JA, Thompson JD (Eds). TeLinde's Operative Gynecology, 8th edition. Philadelphia, PA, USA: Lippincott-Raven Publishers; 1997. pp. 687-729.

CASE 77: VAGINAL HYSTERECTOMY AS EMERGENCY PROCEDURE FOR CORNUAL ECTOPIC PREGNANCY

Name: Ms. YM
Age: 41 years
Parity: 2 FT (full term) SVD (spontaneous vaginal delivery)
Indication for surgery: Cornual ectopic pregnancy.
Medical/surgical comorbidity: None
Operative time: 90 minutes (inclusive of cystoscopy and uterosacral colposuspension).
Hemoglobin pre- and postoperative: 12.5 g/dL, 12.3 g/dL
Recovery course: Discharge day 1, no analgesics, return to work within 1 week.
Pathology report: Benign oviducts, 80 g uterus with left corneal ectopic pregnancy [add 10% to uterine weight, specimen sent directly in formalin to pathology. Gross weight directly in operation room (OR) would be 10–15% more].
Preoperative evaluation: Patient presented emergency room (ER) with pain and was found to have an 8 cm craniocaudal uterus with 7 week left cornual ectopic and fetal cardiac activity. There was no evidence of internal bleeding. Vitals were stable. Patient expressed that pregnancy was unplanned and that her fertility was completed. In light of this vaginal hysterectomy (VH) was offered as alternative to laparotomy with cornual resection. Patient readily accepted this offer.
Surgery: Examination under anesthesia revealed freely mobile uterus. Cervix with traction descended to hymen, indicative of a prolapse Grade 2. Surgical help and hysterectomy instruments were not available. Surgeon used vaginoplasty instruments and assisted by a scrub nurse with no surgical assistant training. These factors prolonged the operative time; however, the hysterectomy proceeded without incident and minimal blood loss. Uterus and cervix delivered as single specimen, and marked dilated but unruptured left cornua was noted. Adnexae were easily visualized and accessed for prophylactic salpingectomy. Uterosacral high colposuspension with subsequent cystoscopy completed the operation.

LESSONS

- This was clearly the right decision for this patient. Laparotomy with cornual excision is an invasive operation with greater potential for blood loss and risks of uterine rupture in subsequent pregnancy. VH was an easier operation to perform, with much lower risk for patient morbidity in both present and future. Permanent sterility as consequence of the surgery was an additional benefit to this patient as per her wishes.
- Cystoscopy was performed in this case due to the added colposuspension. Cystoscopy as routine in VH is highly debatable in terms of cost benefit because ureter injury risk is extremely low. However, when the surgeon after completing VH performs a high colposuspension, ureter injury risk is very real, and particularly of kinking variety. Such injuries can easily and immediately be resolved without sequela by simply cutting the offending suture. Routine cystoscopy is thus a must when doing such cases.

CASE 78: VAGINAL SUPRACERVICAL HYSTERECTOMY 10 YEARS AFTER MESH HYSTEROPEXY

Name: Ms. DB
Age: 53 years
Parity: 2 FT VD
Indication for surgery: Menometrorrhagia and endometrial hyperplasia.
Medical/surgical comorbidity: Abdominosacral mesh hysteropexy with bilateral paravaginal repair. Vertical laparotomy scar.
Operative time: 2 hours 30 minutes
Hemoglobin pre- and postoperative: 13 g/dL, 11.8 g/dL
Recovery course: Discharged from recovery, no postoperative pain, no analgesics.
Pathology report: 70 g uterus, endometrial complex hyperplasia.
Preoperative evaluation: Patient had 2 years of irregular bleeding and multiple biopsies. Her symptoms persist, her lining is markedly thickened, she has family history of gynecologic cancer and she thus strongly desired definitive approach with hysterectomy. Uterus was 9-week size and mobile. The cervix was somewhat elongated and prolapsed to a Baden Walker Grade 2. However, she remained asymptomatic from the prolapse surgery she had 10 years prior. A total VH would likely undermine the mesh repair and promote a prolapse recurrence. Patient consented to "Trial Supracervical VH".
What deters/dissuades: Challenge of needing to access anterior peritoneal reflection without dividing pedicles, and then somehow anteflex fundus through anterior colpotomy.

Surgery: Anterior colpotomy was easily achieved, but bleeding was encountered from cervical branch of uterine on patient's left. Compression, cauterization and suture did not achieve complete hemostasis, but reduced bleeding to a slow persistent ooze.

0-prolene stay sutures were used to "walk up the uterus" and flip fundus through the colpotomy. This maneuver fully achieved tamponade of the cervical bleeder. Clamp, cut and suture techniques were utilized to sequentially divided all lateral pedicles in top-down fashion from utero-ovarian to uterine artery. At this point the uterine body was amputated from cervix. Left uterine artery bleeding was somewhat brisk, but uterine artery is not inclined to retract from view. With uterine specimen removed, visualization was quite good. Long-weighted speculum was inserted over cervix into pelvis, and the bleeder rather easily identified and secured with suture. An 11-number blade was used to perform a reverse top-down cervical conization to remove residual endometrium. Cervical defect was then sutured, copious irrigation confirmed pelvic hemostasis, and the anterior vaginal epithelium was sutured back on to cervix.

LESSON

- Supracervical VH is feasible in select patients. Uterus must be small enough (12-week size or less) for anterior peritoneum to be readily accessible and for fundus to be feasibly deliverable through that colpotomy.

CASE 79: VAGINAL HYSTERECTOMY (VH): INCARCERATED PROLAPSE DUE TO CERVICAL LEIOMYOMA AND AN INTRAMURAL MYOMA

Name: Ms. Y
Age: 54
Parity: G2p1011
Last delivery: Remote
Complaint: 2-month history of protrusion from vaginal opening with inability to reduce prolapse and pelvic/abdominal pain.
History: Prior to presentation, the patient presented to her local rural Emergency Department with cyclic 9/10 pain in the pelvis, some discharge and light bleeding. No significant medical comorbidities.
Physical examination: Complete uterovaginal prolapse (Baden Walker 14/44/40) with a large cervical mass that prevented reduction of the prolapse. Patient was in considerable pain and was unable to sit due to the protrusion. She was forced to stand or lie down only.
Course: Patient was directly admitted to the hospital for bed rest, computed tomography (CT) scan, and surgery. CT immediately after admission showed: a uterine prolapse with an ulcerated mass in the cervix measuring approximately 5.5 cm × 7.0 cm × 3.9 cm. The uterus measured approximately 7.1 cm × 7.4 cm × 18 cm [anteroposterior (AP), transverse, longitudinal] including the prolapsed cervical mass. There was a 5.5 cm × 6.0 cm × 5.3 cm soft tissue mass in the fundus that appeared predominantly intramural and showed a submucosal component. A right hydroureteronephrosis was noted; a normal creatinine was reassuring.
Interpretation: Incarcerated prolapse in a clinical setting of two myomata, one in the cervix and second in the fundus, resulted in complete immobilization of the uterus in a complete procidentia (Fig. 1).
Treatment course: Cervical myomectomy, diagnostic cystoureteroscopy and diagnostic hysteroscopy were chosen as the initial treatments in order to relieve pressure and obtain a diagnosis of the cervical mass. After resection of the cervical fibroid, hysteroscopy revealed a submucous myoma, no attempt was made to resect that lesion.

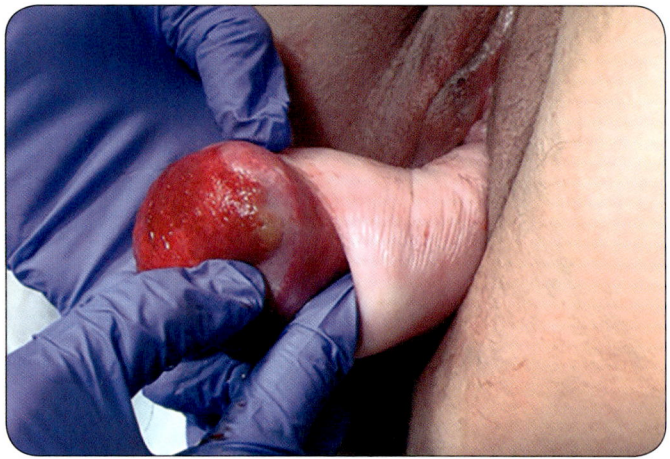

Fig. 1: Demonstration of large cervical myoma in operating theater prior to myomectomy.

Cystoureteroscopy revealed patency of both ureters. Pathology report indicated an 8 cm bland spindle cell myoma. Resection of the myoma resulted in the ability to reduce the prolapse with relief of the cyclic uterine pain and abdominal pain. She was discharged for return to the clinic. Approximately 4 weeks later, the patient underwent vaginal hysterectomy using standard technique. Speciman 292 g with no morcellation needed. Pathology showed a 6 cm intramural fundal leiomyoma.

Postoperative visit revealed normalized, gastrointestinal and genitourinary function with internalization of the apex of the vagina.

LESSON

- An urgent clinical presentation may require staging of treatment into two separate operations. Resection of the cervical myoma resulted in relief of pain in a setting where hydroureteronephrosis was developing. After stabilization of the patient and pathological analysis of her tumor, a routine vaginal hysterectomy was performed.

CASE 80: VH IN NULLIPARA WITH ONGOING CHEMOTHERAPY FOR NON-GYNECOLOGIC MALIGNANCIES

Name: Ms. L
Age: 43 years
Parity: G 0
Last childbirth: N/A
Complaint: Referred by Medical Oncology Service due to persistent vaginal bleeding.
History: Colorectal cancer treated surgically, with chemotherapy, and radiation. Currently being treated with chemotherapy and she was status post-stem cell transplant for *Myelodysplastic Syndrome*. Anemia and thrombocytopenia does complicate ability to tolerate current oncology treatments. At the time of presentation, patient was receiving blood and platelet transfusions at 2-week intervals.
Interpretation: Very small descent uterus in a medically compromised patient with persistent bleeding that necessitated frequent blood and platelet transfusions. Patient needed minimally invasive vaginal approach for contemplated surgery in order to minimize surgical recovery and complications.
Course: Two months prior to the definitive procedure a hysteroscopy and dilation and curettage (D&C) were negative for pathology but failed to decrease bleeding. Bleeding persisted. Vaginal hysterectomy was recommended and cleared with her medical oncologist/stem cell transplant physician.
Treatment: Vaginal hysterectomy and cystoureteroscopy were performed after 3 packets of platelets and 3 units of packed red blood cells. Presenting packed cell volume was 21% and platelet count 74,000. Because of the very small size of the uterus, traditional clamps (Zeppelin and Heaney) could not be used effectively. For that reason, a small pedicle sealing device normally used in intestinal surgery was used to perform the procedure. Nulliparous state restricted vaginal access to the uterus; however, the small pedicle sealing device permitted successful access to one pedicle at a time, while taking care not to take large bites. The postoperative course was uncomplicated. Discharged to home on hospital day 2.
Pathology report: Uterus and cervix: cervix with no significant histopathologic change; leiomyoma; inactive endometrium; negative for malignancy. 16-g uterus. Uterine measurements: 5 cm-superior inferior, 2.7 cm-transverse diameter and 2.5 cm-AP (Fig. 1).

Postoperative examination revealed ongoing treatment for myelodysplastic syndrome, no vaginal bleeding, and no complications associated with her hysterectomy.

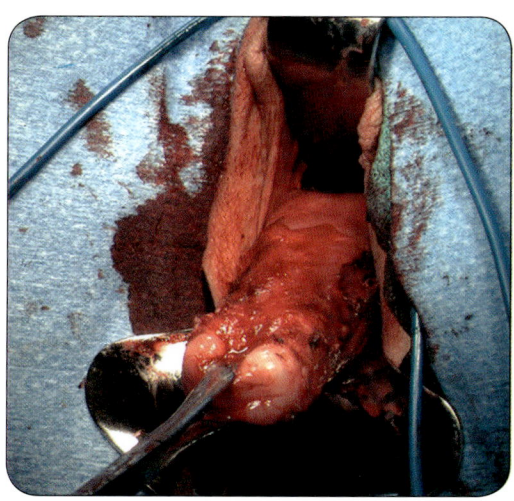

Fig. 1: Nulliparous, undescended and very small uterus immediately prior to transection of the adnexal pedicles. Note the location of the anterior peritoneal fold.

LESSON

- Vaginal hysterectomy can be complicated by size. Most emphasis has been addressed to the enlarged uterus; however, the very small uterus can also be problematic. Special techniques, such as the pedicle sealing device, can be useful. The surgeon should be alert to very small pedicles as large bites exposes vulnerable anatomy to damage.

CASE 81: VH FOR ENDOMETRIAL CARCINOMA IN MORBIDLY OBESE WITH HISTORY OF CAESAREAN SECTION

Name: Ms. W
Age: 58 years
Parity: G1p1001
Last delivery: Remote
Complaint: Recent onset postmenopausal uterine bleeding followed by endometrial biopsy showing endometrial adenocarcinoma.
History: Referred by gynecologic oncology for consideration of vaginal hysterectomy due to inability of patient to tolerate full-staging surgical procedure through the abdomen or endoscopically. Multiple medical comorbidities include morbid obesity [weight 141 kg, 311 lbs, body mass index (BMI) 59], diabetes [peripheral neuropathy, albuminuria, glycosylated hemoglobin (HbA_{1c}) prior to surgery 10.2% which is significantly elevated and in a range that impairs healing, especially in large abdominal incisions], obstructed sleep apnea [using continuous positive airway pressure (CPAP)] and hypertension. She is unable to lie flat for any significant period of time.
Physical examination: Morbid obesity with multiple abdominal folds (pannus), ptosis of the mons pubis, deep narrow vagina with palpable cervix, and some vertical mobility.
Interpretation: Morbidly obese and medically compromised patient in whom the risks of vaginal hysterectomy (incomplete staging) are less than the risks of a complete staging procedure due to inability to tolerate the surgical burden.
Treatment course: Admitted for hysterectomy. Vaginal hysterectomy performed. Valuable techniques included elevation of the pannus with taping procedure prior to the surgery (Fig. 1); uterosacral massage with traction prior to incision; clamping and transection of uterosacral, cardinal and bladder pillars prior to attempt to dissect caesarean section scar; and use of the broad ligament space of Sheth to outflank and isolate the Caesarean Section scar prior to lysis of the scar.

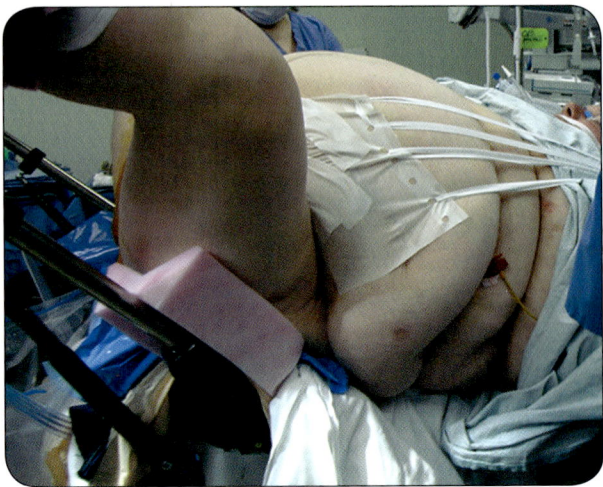

Fig. 1: Morbidly obese patient with tape elevation of large pannus and foam padding to protect vulnerable pressure points in the lower extremities. Elevation of the pannus significantly increases exposure of the vaginal vault and enhances the ability of the surgeon to operate efficiently.

Pathology report: Uterus: endometrial adenocarcinoma endometrioid type, FIGO Grade 1, negative for myometrial invasion, arising in a background of complex atypical hyperplasia involving adenomyosis; multiple leiomyomata, largest measuring 19 mm; separate benign endometrial polyp; uterine cervix with no significant histopathologic changes. Uterine weight 151 g.

Postoperatively the patient did well with no complications and has required no further treatment for her cancer.

LESSON

- In a difficult vaginal hysterectomy, preoperative preparation, e.g. maximizing exposure for successful surgery, is very important. A challenging vaginal case may be in the patient's best interest, given medical comorbidities.

Index

Note: Page numbers followed by *f* refer to figure.

A

Abdominal hernioplasty 100
Abdominal hysterectomy 5, 57
Abdominal LNR for endometrial CA 102
Abdominal omentectomy 70
Abdominosacral mesh hysteropexy 139
Abnormal uterine bleeding 39
Accessible cervix 22
Adenoacanthoma 93
Adenocarcinoma 70
Adenomyosis 142
Adenomyotic uterine walls 126
Adhesions of omentum to abdominal wall 117
Adnexal malignancy 46
Adnexal mass 64
Adnexal pathology 29, 73
Allis' forceps 43*f*, 67
Altered uterocervical angle 110
Anemia 54, 141
Anterior colporrhaphy 134
Anterior myoma 22
Anterior peritoneum 37
Anterior vaginal mucosa 43*f*
Asherman's syndrome 48
Atrophic endometrium 134

B

Babcock's forceps 31*f*, 44*f*, 64
Basal hyperplasia 32
Benign endometrial biopsy 22, 25, 117, 119
Benign mobile ovarian cyst for adnexectomy 10
Benign ovarian fibroma 46
Benign ovarian fibrothecoma 69
Benign oviducts 115, 119
Bicornuate uterus 135
Bilateral hydrosalpinx in a nullipara 60
Bilateral large hydrosalpinx 81
Bilateral pelvic lymphadenectomy 113
Bilateral salpingo-oophorectomy 13
Black silk traction sutures 43*f*
Bladder injury 40
Bladder retractor 13, 42, 77
Bladder stone 136
Blood transfusion 8, 30
Brenner tumor 68
Broad ligament fibroid 71*f*
Broad ligament myomectomy 71

C

Caesarean sections 29
Cardinal ligament pedicle 54
Cervical intraepithelial neoplasia (CIN) III 126
Cervical leiomyoma 140
Cervicouterine junction 120
Cervicouterine surface 30*f*
Cervix 13
Cervix with physiological descent 107
Chocolate fluid 116
Clear cell carcinoma 87
Colorectal cancer 141
Complex hyperplasia 92
Complex hyperplasia plus focal endometrial "CA" 100
Concomitant salpingo-oophorectomy 69
Contralateral endometriotic cyst 125
Contralateral hemihysterectomized uterus 4
Contralateral salpingo-oophorectomy 95
Cornual area 42
Corpus cancer syndrome 96, 98
Corpus luteum 59
Cuff removal 88
Cul-de-sac peritoneum 116
Cysto-rectoceles 136

D

Deaver's retractor 109*f*
Debulking of adenomyotic uterine walls 80
Debulking of thick uterine 9*f*
Diabetic with endometrial cancer 82
Diagnostic laparoscopy 29
Dimple sign 37
Dysfunctional uterine bleeding 123
Dysmenorrhea 54

E

Ectopic pregnancy 49
Endometrial ablation 39
Endometrial biopsy 93
Endometrial cancer 29, 93*f*
Endometrial complex hyperplasia with atypia 98
Endometrial complex hyperplasia without atypia 101
Endometrial HP study 93
Endometrial hyperplasia 30, 139
Endometrioid adenocarcinoma 41, 82, 93
Endometriosis of ovary 58
Endometriotic cyst 80, 111
Endometriotic cystectomy 65
Endometriotic ovarian cyst 59
Endometrium 13
External cervical OS 89
Extraperitoneal subcervical tunneling 67

F

Failed abdominal hysterectomy 130
Failed trial vaginal route 96
Fair amount of vesicles 128
Fallopian tube 58
Fibroid for enucleation 112, 115
Fibrothecoma with benign endometrial polyp 69
Flimsy adhesions 131
Focal endometrioid adenocarcinoma 100
Fundal fibroid 11
Fundus of the uterus 109

G

Genital tract 39, 123

H

Hemihysterectomized uterus 37, 57
Hemorrhagic cyst 129
Hemostasis 13
Hydatidiform mole 128
Hydrosalpinx 37, 57, 60
Hysterectomies in nullipara 61
Hysterectomized uterus 82, 99
Hysterectomy with unilateral salpingo-oophorectomy 91

I

Inaccessible adnexa 54
Incarcerated prolapse 140
Incisional hernia repair 100
Infundibulopelvic ligament 57, 129
International federation of gynecology and obstetrics (FIGO) grade II 102
Intramural myoma 140
Intramyometrial coring 47
Intrauterine device 39
Intrauterine morcellation 116
IV sodium pentothal 133

K

Kilogram uterus 21

L

Laparoscopic adhesiolysis of "band" 107
Laparoscopically-assisted vaginal hysterectomy for large uterus with adnexal pathology 58
Laparoscopic cholecystectomy 102
Laparoscopic hysterectomy 58
Laparoscopic surgery 87, 88
Laparotomy with cornual excision 138
Large bilateral hydrosalpinx 60
Large-sized uterus 112
Lateral vaginal walls 41
Left ovarian endometriotic cyst 35, 63
Left ovarian ligament 49
Leiomyoma 54
Leiomyomata 34
Lithotomy 101
Lower pole of fibroid 13
Lymphadenectomy 59, 91
Lymph node 59
Lymph nodes removal 70, 88

M

Mackendrot's ligament 110, 134
Maylard incision 53
Menometrorrhagia 139
Menorrhagia 54
Menstrual hygiene 77
Mesoovarium 57
Metastatic breast cancer 127
Minilaparotomy 117
Minimal invasive surgery 117
Mobile uterus 22
Morcellation 5
Multiple leiomyomata 142
Myelodysplastic syndrome 141
Myometrial invasion 82

N

Necrotic collapsed benign cyst 129
Nullipara with intact hymen 77
Nulliparity plus endometriotic cyst 80

O

Obese cigarette smoker 49
Obese patient 35
Obstetric trauma 78
Omentectomy 59
Omentectomy with bilateral pelvic lymphadenectomy 70
Operation theater/room (OT/OR) for hysteroscopy 41
Ovarian adenocarcinoma 70
Ovarian cyst 57
Ovarian cystectomy 30, 34
Ovarian dermoid/teratoma 58
Ovarian endometriosis with positive "dimple sign" 111
Ovarian malignancy 70, 113
Ovarian teratoma 64

P

Para-colic gutters 70, 113
Parametrial infiltration 133
Parasitic myoma and inaccessible adnexa 120
Paratubal cysts 34
Pelvic inflammatory disease 116
Pelvic lymph nodes 59
Pelvic pathology 123
Pelvic ultrasound 49
Peritoneal cavity 70, 113
Peritoneal edge 46
Peritoneal fluid 93
Peritoneal wash for cytology 59
Pfannenstiel's incision 96
Posterior colpoperineorrhaphy 134
Posterior fornix 64
Postmenopausal bleeding and endometrial histopathology 87
Postmenopause atrophy of IP ligaments 54
Post-uterine artery division 120
Pouch of Douglas 4, 29
Preliminary twilight sleep 133
Proliferative endometrium 49
Prophylactic oophorectomy 58
Prophylactic salpingectomy 58
Prophylactic salpingo-oophorectomy 29
Pryor's technique 11*f*
Ptosis of the mons pubis 142
Pubic bone 120
Pubic symphysis 108
Pudendal and paracervical nerve blocks 132
Pulmonary fibrosis 132

R

Rectal trauma 111
Rectouterine peritoneum 100
Recurrent postmenopause bleeding 24
Reddish brown cyst 129
Retroflexion of the uterus 66
Retroverted and retroflexed uterus 38
Right hemi-uterus 49
Role of sonography-n-sonologist 59
Round ligament 57s
Rupture uterus 29

S

Salpingo-oophorectomy at vaginal hysterectomy 87
Salpingo-oophorectomy of contralateral side 91, 93
Scar tissue 53
Schuchardt's incision 77
Serous cell carcinoma 87
Severe adenomyosis 34
Sheth adnexa clamp 63*f*
Simple hyperplasia 92
Simple serous cyst 58
Sim's speculum 77
Sim's vaginal speculum 63*f*
Sizeable endometriotic cyst 36
Small blood vessels 58
Solid ovarian tumor 68
Squamous metaplasia 32
Square metaplasia 93
Stress urinary incontinence (SUI) repair 32
Surgery of laparotomy 87
Suspected adenomyosis 49

T

Technique of morcellation 22
Tenaculum traction 49
Thrombocytopenia 141
Total uterine bisection 4
Transabdominal pelvic sonography 109*f*
Transvaginal obturator tape 32
Transverse rectus muscle 117
Trial vaginal hysterectomy (VH) case 107
Trial vaginal route 35
Tubal hydrosalpinx 37
Tubal sterilization 47

Tubes and ovaries 131
Twisted gangrenous cystic mass 73
Twisted ovarian cyst 73*f*, 129

U

Unanticipated uterine adhesions 117
Undiagnosed uteroabdominal band 107
Unilateral salpingo-oophorectomy 82
Urinary catheter 136
Uterine adenomyosis 30
Uterine bulk 54
Uterine conservation 127
Uterine debulking 3
    method (technique) 3
Uterine fibroids 8, 71
Uterine fibroids with bicornuate uterus 135
Uterine fundus 109
Uterine malignancy 87
Uterine pathology 22
Uterine prolapse with cystocele 136
Uterine tissue 120
Uterine vessels 8, 13
Uterocervical adhesions with abdominal wall 108
Uterocervical angle 66
Uterocervical-broad ligament 30*f*, 37
Uterocervical junction 38, 66*f*
Uterosacral colpo suspension 49, 117, 118
Uterosacral descent 46
Uterosacral ligament pedicle 46
Uterus with dense fundus 117

V

Vaginal cuff 41, 120
Vaginal delivery 118
Vaginal hysterectomy 5, 9
Vaginal hysterectomy (VH) with uterine debulking 8
Vaginal hysterectomy with vaginal cuff 82
Vaginal morcellation techniques 22
Vaginal route for hysterectomy 124
Vaginal supracervical hysterectomy 139
Vaginal wall retractors 77
Vascular uterine walls 128
Veere's needle 57, 64
Vertical laparotomy 46
Vertical sub-umbilical incision 88
Vertical suprapubic incision 59
Vesicouterine peritoneum 100, 123
Vesicouterine space 53
VH with bilateral salpingectomy 80
Vulva vaginal area 96*f*

W

Wedge resection 120
Well-differentiated endometrial adenocarcinoma 99

Z

Zero spillage 65